The Astrologer's Diet Book

The Astrologer's Diet Book

TERI KING

drawings by Maggie Ragner

ALLISON & BUSBY
LONDON

First published in Great Britain 1977 by
Allison & Busby Limited, 6a Noel Street, London W1V 3RB

Copyright © Teri King 1977

ISBN 0 85031 193 4

*Set in 10 on 11 point Times
and printed by Villiers Publications Ltd,
Ingestre Road, London*

CONTENTS

To my children
Deborah, Justin and Lindsay

Introduction

Astrology can be as invaluable in assessing a person's physical tendencies as it is in understanding other aspects of the personality; it must always be remembered, however, that each individual will be influenced specifically by the hour, day, year and place of his or her birth. Because astrology is such a complex science, it is of course only possible for a book like this to be a general guide, and in order to work out what is known as an individual's birth-chart an astrologer must have access to specific personal details.

It cannot be denied that most people are happiest when they are slim and healthy, and the main purpose of this book is to give the reader, first, enough information about the natural inclinations of members of each sign—general characteristics, emotional outlook, physical types, health hazards—to be able to identify and predict the likely causes of overweight; and, secondly, advice and common-sense suggestions on the most effective ways for each sign to cope with weight problems, together with useful fashion tips that bear in mind the physical tendencies of different signs.

For each birth sign, the possible associated nutritional deficiencies are specified, and details are given of the right kinds of food to make up for any lack. Then there are special recipes geared towards individual signs; some of these are not directly part of a slimming diet but are designed simply to bring out the best in members of that sign—and this in itself can be a big step in the right direction, for often the need to overeat is linked with feeling depressed and under the weather. Each sign then has a Special Seven-Day Diet, carefully tailored to the emotional and physical needs of its subjects. Then there is a more exotic recipe or two chosen from countries ruled by each sign. The quiz at the end of each section will help you determine what shape you're in (if you don't already know!) and whether you're heading for weight problems.

General points about slimming

The first thing to do is to take a good long look at yourself (prefer-ably wearing very little) in a full-length mirror. Forget about "vital statistics"; this fashionable but ridiculously deceptive way of des-cribing female proportions is no real indication of beauty and health. Half a dozen women of the same height and identical measurements will all have bodies which appear quite different to the onlooker, since these measurements take no account of bone structure, the set of shoulders, thickness of chest, legs and thighs or padding in other parts. So check your height and weight against the tables on page 10 before deciding you are overweight.

If you're still not sure, or if you just dread standing on the weighing scales to find out, there is another way to estimate and calculate fat. Excess fat accumulates on various parts of the body and is noticeable under the skin, so a rough but fairly reliable test is to pinch your skin between finger and thumb. If there is no fat, the amount lifted should be less than a quarter of an inch. Fat is starting to accumulate when half an inch thick can be gathered. But if the piece lifted is three-quarters of an inch or even an inch thick, then that portion is too fat.

To slim successfully you need three main things: motivation, information and willpower. The motivation might well be health: there are some complaints which fat people are more prone to than thin people (heart conditions, kidney diseases, diabetes, digestive disorders). When you've worked out how much overweight you are, fill a suitcase until it weighs as much as your surplus fat; try carrying it up and down the stairs a few times and you'll understand why being fat puts so much extra strain on your body.

The most important information you need is about calories. Your calorie intake varies depending on the sort of person you are and the life you lead (and as you get older, from about the age of twenty-five, you tend to need fewer calories). One person may use up 4,000 calories in energy a day, while another may need less than 2,000. It is when your calorific intake exceeds your daily energy needs that unwanted fat begins to accumulate. The Calorie Expenditure Chart on page 162 will give you some idea of how many calories an hour are burned up by various activities. The Calorie Tables of basic foods on pages 163-8 will help you regulate your eating (remember that calorie values depend on the method of cooking, so if for instance butter is used for frying, then the appropriate number of additional calories must be included). It is generally reckoned that the average slimmer, in order to see results, should restrict calorie intake to between 1,000 and 1,500 calories per day. With this in mind, most of the meals specified in this book have a calorific value of between 250-500 calories each; obviously it is impossible to be exact about "medium portions" and so on, so it's ultimately up to you to be sensible in assessing and balancing your own daily needs.

Of course, it's impossible to cut off the outside world simply because you're on a diet. So if you're asked out to a sumptuous banquet and suffer a temporary loss of willpower, whatever you do don't just sit about the next day feeling guilty about it. Guilt is one of the surest ways to drive yourself to seek consolation in food. There is absolutely no need to despair, and instead a bit of constructive action should immediately be taken. Follow the One-Day Hangover Diet or the One-Day Beauty Diet on page 15, and this will quickly help repair the damage done the night before. After this carry on your diet from where you left off. One break won't put back all the excess fat already lost. Another way of dealing with irresistible invitations to dinner is to cut down what you eat for a couple of days before the event, so that you have some extra calories for the day when you are certain to exceed your limit.

Your problem, if you're a certain type, may on the other hand be underweight, in which case the Menus for Skinnies on pages 11-14 are specially for you.

If you're more than just a couple of pounds overweight, the ideal technique is to set yourself a target and phase your weight loss over a number of weeks, rather than going on a brutal crash diet one week only to return to your normal overeating the next. The Special Seven-Day Diets should be repeated, and varied as suggested, as often as necessary, until your desired weight is reached — and then you must continue to eat sensibly. If you have any particular health problems, it is always wise to check with your doctor before embarking on any radical dieting.

Above all, be honest with yourself—don't kid yourself that you're eating less than you are. If you honestly do want to lose weight, the only way to do it is to eat less, and the aim of this book is to show members of each sign of the zodiac the most painless and compatible ways of succeeding.

HEIGHT AND WEIGHT TABLES
Desirable weights for men and women of age 25 and over as ordinarily dressed

MEN

Height feet	inches	Small frame pounds	Medium frame pounds	Large frame pounds
5	2	116–125	124–133	131–142
5	3	119–128	127–136	133–144
5	4	122–132	130–140	137–149
5	5	126–136	134–144	141–153
5	6	129–139	137–147	145–157
5	7	133–143	141–151	149–162
5	8	136–147	145–156	153–166
5	9	140–151	149–160	157–170
5	10	144–155	153–164	161–174
5	11	148–159	157–168	165–180
6	0	152–180	161–172	169–184
6	1	157–169	166–179	174–189
6	2	163–174	171–184	179–196
6	3	168–180	176–189	184–202
6	4	172–184	180–195	188–210

WOMEN

Height feet	inches	Small frame pounds	Medium frame pounds	Large frame pounds
4	11	104–111	110–118	117–127
5	0	105–113	112–120	119–129
5	1	107–115	114–122	121–131
5	2	110–118	117–125	124–135
5	3	113–121	120–128	127–138
5	4	116–125	124–135	133–145
5	5	119–128	127–138	138–150
5	6	123–132	130–140	142–154
5	7	126–136	134–144	145–158
5	8	129–139	137–147	149–162
5	9	133–143	141–151	152–166
5	10	136–147	145–155	155–169
5	11	139–150	148–158	159–173
6	0	143–155	152–164	163–178

MENUS FOR SKINNIES

It is better to be a little underweight than overweight. On the other hand, a bit of padding in the right places looks good and helps to keep you healthy and warm. If skinniness is your problem it is important to eat larger amounts of those foods which keep you relaxed, for tension is often what prevents people from gaining sufficient weight. Practically all vitamins and minerals are needed for such relaxation, but calcium and vitamin D are of special significance. Here is a week's diet which will help considerably.

Monday

Breakfast: 1 large glass sweet fruit juice
cereal with cream
1 glass vitamin D milk, or coffee (half cream)

Mid-morning: 1 banana whipped into a glass milk, or 1 yogurt
1,000 units vitamin D yeast concentrate

Lunch: 2 scrambled eggs
wholewheat toast with plenty of butter
fruit salad
1 glass milk

Mid-afternoon: 1 tablespoon black molasses or honey in 1 glass
milk / 1 ripe banana whipped into 1 glass pineapple juice

Dinner: Hot soup
liver and bacon
spinach sprinkled with olive oil
apple pie and cream
1 coffee (half cream)

Before retiring: 1 tablespoon brewers' yeast in 1 yogurt

Tuesday

Breakfast: 1 glass pineapple juice
cereal with cream sprinkled with wheatgerm and
dates
1 glass milk, or coffee (half cream)

Mid-morning: 1 banana whipped into glass of milk, or yogurt, or
carrot juice
1,000 units vitamin D yeast concentrate

Lunch: Chopped egg and celery salad with lemon and olive-
                 oil dressing
                 toasted rye bread, with butter
                 1 glass milk with black molasses
Mid-afternoon: Ripe banana whipped into milk
Dinner: Boiled or grilled fish
                 stewed tomatoes
                 baked potato
                 green salad with lemon and olive oil dressing
                 baked apple with cream
                 coffee (half cream)

Wednesday

Breakfast: 1 large glass orange juice
                 1 boiled egg
                 2 slices toast with butter
                 1 glass milk or creamy coffee
Mid-morning: 1 banana whipped into milk or yogurt
                 1,000 units vitamin D yeast concentrate
Lunch: Tuna fish and celery salad with lemon and olive oil
                 dressing
                 rye bread
                 1 glass milk flavoured with honey
Mid-afternoon: 1 banana whipped into milk
Dinner: Chopped cabbage and raisin salad with sour cream
                 dressing or mayonnaise
                 chopped steak mixed with wheatgerm and parsley
                 stewed apricots and cream
                 coffee (half cream)

Thursday

Breakfast: Cooked cereal with wheatgerm, honey and cream
                 wholewheat toast with butter
                 1 glass vitamin D milk, or coffee (half cream)
Mid-morning: 1 banana whipped into glass of milk or 1 yogurt
                 1,000 units vitamin D yeast concentrate
Lunch: Large fruit salad sprinkled with nuts
                 wholewheat biscuits
                 1 glass yogurt with cinnamon and honey
Mid-afternoon: 1 banana whipped into pineapple juice or milk
Dinner: Green salad with lemon and olive oil dressing
                 beef Stroganoff/grilled steak/lamb chop

            buttered green beans
            apple pie
            lemon tea with honey, or coffee (half cream)
Before retiring: 1 tablespoon brewers' yeast stirred into yogurt

Friday

Breakfast: Stewed apricots
            crisp bacon
            wholewheat toast with butter
            1 glass milk, or coffee (half cream)
Mid-morning: 1 banana whipped into 1 glass milk or yogurt
Lunch: Cottage cheese salad with pears or pineapple
            cream crackers
            1 glass milk or coffee made half with cream
Mid-afternoon: 1 tablespoon molasses in milk / 1 banana whipped
                into pineapple juice
Dinner: Steak and onions
            cauliflower sprinkled with wheatgerm and browned
              in butter
            cucumber salad
            baked custard
            coffee (half cream)

Saturday

Breakfast: 1 large glass orange juice
            scrambled eggs
            muffin with butter and honey
            1 glass milk
Mid-morning: 1 banana whipped into milk or yogurt
Lunch: Pancakes with sugar and butter
            fresh or stewed fruit
            1 glass milk
Mid-afternoon: 1 banana whipped into milk or coffee made half
                with cream
Dinner: Tomato juice
            liver and onions
            cauliflower sprinkled with cheese
            potato in jacket
            sliced banana with cream
            lemon tea with honey, or coffee (half cream)

Sunday

Breakfast:	Honey and apricots wholewheat toast with butter crisp bacon 1 glass milk
Mid-morning:	1 banana whipped into milk or yogurt 1,000 units vitamin D yeast concentrate
Lunch:	Stuffed tomato with cottage cheese, wheatgerm and celery wholewheat bread 1 glass vitamin D milk with honey
Mid-afternoon:	1 banana whipped into milk or yogurt coffee made half with cream
Dinner:	Cold meat, with cranberry sauce coleslaw with cream dressing roast or baked potato in jacket
Before retiring:	1 tablespoon brewers' yeast in milk or yogurt

ONE-DAY HANGOVER DIET

Do you have bloodshot eyes? Does your mouth taste like the bottom of a bird-cage? Then try this one-day kind-to-your-stomach diet.

Breakfast:	1 large glass orange or grapefruit juice
	2 cups lemon tea with honey, or 1 cup black coffee
Mid-morning:	1 large glass celery or carrot or apple juice (or all three combined); if no fresh vegetable juice is available drink orange or grapefruit juice instead
Lunch:	2 cups hot soup
	1 yogurt with cinnamon, nutmeg or honey
Mid-afternoon:	1 glass vegetable or fruit juice (as mid-morning choice)
Dinner:	1 cup tomato soup or tomato juice
	1 glass yogurt with cinnamon, nutmeg or honey
	1 cup black coffee or lemon tea

ONE-DAY BEAUTY DIET

After too much feasting, when you begin to feel stuffy or when your clothes begin to stick out in the wrong places, try this painless one-day diet.

Breakfast:	1 sliced orange or ½ grapefruit
	1 cup black coffee, if you must, but herb tea preferable
Mid-morning:	1 glass fruit juice (anything except banana)
Lunch:	Chopped carrot and cottage cheese on a few lettuce leaves sprinkled with lemon juice
	1 cup light vegetable soup, or mint tea
Mid-afternoon:	1 glass any fruit juice except banana
Dinner:	Spinach sprinkled with lemon
	fresh fruit salad
	yogurt
	black coffee
Before retiring:	Still hungry? Then more fruit juice or lemon tea.

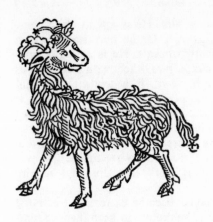

Aries (the ram)

The sign of the warrior or pioneer

March 21—April 20

The first fire sign:	Energetic, enthusiastic, impulsive, positive, enterprising, lives in the mind
Ruler: Mars	**Gems:** Amethyst, diamond
Colour: Red	**Metal:** Iron

GENERAL CHARACTERISTICS

Are you wilful, impatient and headstrong? Do others depend on you for leadership and advice? Do you fail to learn from past mistakes? If so, the chances are that your birth sign is Aries.

Those born under this sign are fiery and brilliant, with a great sense of adventure and an aggressive, pioneering spirit. They seize upon new ideas, and have the practicality and daring to realise their ambitions. The only problem is that when the Arietian is unable to find a sympathetic ear or to develop a plan immediately, other ideas soon become equally interesting. In other words, this type is inconsistent and not particularly good at seeing tasks through; once an obstacle is encountered the project concerned is usually shelved.

The Arietian man likes to be in a position of authority, to be a trail-blazer and have others follow him. He is apt to leave home early to establish a family of his own. Or he may start his own business; freelance work frequently appeals. He is eternally optimistic and young in spirit, and can inspire others with a contagious enthusiasm. One of his faults, however, is a tendency to want everything his own way; independence to the point of rashness is another characteristic. The Arietian is impulsive, often flying headlong into a situation before investigating its dangers and possibilities sufficiently; he may have cause to regret such spur-of-the-moment action. Furthermore, he tends to overestimate his own abilities, though he is excellent at work that does not require sustained effort.

Those close to the Arietian could become extremely frustrated when trying to share his thoughts; he prefers to keep them to himself unless absolutely sure he will be understood. People may describe this character as selfish, an accusation which isn't without foundation. When he sees something he likes, he rushes in and tries to take it. The person who beats you to the one and only seat left on the train—that was him. He also tears into relationships, and may take his leave in much the same way. The negative Aries type unhappily possesses an excess of the weaker characteristics, pursuing one line of thought one day and another the next. Small wonder then that it's impossible for him to get anything off the ground.

The female of the species displays all the vitality and warmth of her male counterpart. She loathes half-heartedness or want of enthusiasm in those around her; the ultra-scrupulous person who weighs every word and deliberates long over every decision is a terrible trial to her, a feeling she usually makes abundantly clear. In her private life she likes to run the whole show. The opposite sex do not find her easy to please; she invariably attempts to show she can do everything every bit as well as them, if not better. She is no valuer of the male ego. In fact she can get along very well without a man in her life. When a fuse blows in her house, she's not the type to rush out looking for a male to come to her rescue. Nevertheless, once she has committed herself she makes a good and loyal wife.

Famous Arietians: **Pearl Bailey, Baudelaire, Marlon Brando, James Callaghan, Charlie Chaplin, Bette Davis, Doris Day, Alec Guinness, Adolf Hitler, Thomas Jefferson, Nikita Khrushchev, Paul Robeson, Tennessee Williams.**

LOVE, SEX AND THE ARIETIAN

Arietians are rarely short of admirers. They attract others because of their dash and spirit, but while they may please and stimulate they often fail to satisfy. Arietians love by sight; looks are important to them, yet in the final analysis they choose with their head more than with their heart, and the mental qualities of the lover influence the choice to a large extent. They are impulsive emotionally, as in all else, and go after the object of their affection with a single-minded drive. Their method is contradictory: they are passionate and aggressive like the ram one minute, cool and disinterested the next. They also stand ready to fight off the advances of others once they have staked their claim. However they do tend to be more interested in a conquest than in actually settling down. Those born under this sign frequently appear fickle, because they are searching for the ideal love they dream of, and are never content with the imperfect reality.

Arietians are inclined to "wear" the opposite sex—in other words, the partner must be someone whom others can admire. It's important for subjects of Aries to feel they have captured something really worthwhile. Sexually speaking this individual believes that he or she is the most uncomplicated individual in the world. In fact the Arietian's sexual appetite varies quite considerably and usually requires quite a lot of stimulation. While enthusiasm is roused and all is running smoothly, Arietians can relax, and then they suddenly remember that their body and appetites have been neglected for some time. But let one of those gigantic and ambitious schemes bite the dust and the Aries subject is in a sorry state, for when the ego is deflated it takes a while for these types to pick themselves up and start again. In the meantime they become apathetic. Sex loses its appeal, and as a result of disillusionment, inventiveness deserts the Arietian. It is then that they may look for compensation in another direction.

FASHION AND THE ARIETIAN

The typical Arietian realises the value of a good appearance. This type is particular and meticulous in dress at all times. The wardrobe may be sparse, but this individual will inevitably manage to look neat and fresh, even in the oldest of clothes. Those born under this sign will possibly spend a little more on their appearance than can be afforded; they like expensive, well-tailored garments—cheap or shoddy clothes just do not appeal. So there is little clothes advice that can be given to an overweight Arietian. Miss Aries should perhaps be reminded that her favourite bright colours will add a few pounds, whereas darker shades will be more flattering.

For the most part, however, this is an elegant, well-groomed sign; though it might be wise to remember that while it is admirable to keep up with the latest fashion trends, most of them are designed for the "skinny lizzies" displayed in glossy magazines. Overweight Arietians must accept the fact that before they can successfully adopt whatever latest style takes their fancy, it is first necessary to shed those extra pounds. Fortunately this is not an ostentatious sign, and it would be most uncharacteristic for an Aries subject to be caught out in the ridiculous.

PHYSICAL CHARACTERISTICS AND HEALTH

The Arietian man tends to have thick, coarse, curly hair; a long, muscular body with slim hips and broad shoulders; high cheek bones, and a long, straight nose. Not infrequently, in fact, the profile can be compared to that of a ram—no offence meant!

The Aries woman also often has a muscular build, with a thick waistline; a strong face with straight eyebrows, a thin upper lip and highly coloured cheeks; a short neck, and small feet.

Aries rules the head and face, and the planet Mars gives its subjects flaming energy. The personality of this type is intensely alive, the movements quick and impulsive. Too often Arietians make no attempt to control their passions, and more often than not this leads them to commit excesses of one sort or another. There is a marked tendency to overwork the body; many Arietians are careless about their health. They place too much strain on a weak point of their body, or ignore the need to slow down when they are ill. In this way they weaken themselves and aggravate their ailments. Tension may result in headaches and eyestrain. Generally, however, the Arietian is a healthy specimen.

CAUSES OF ARIETIAN OBESITY AND HOW TO COPE

Generally, the Arietian is only a temporary fat person, for overweight is uncharacteristic of this sign. Muscle is more likely than flab. All Arietians are pioneers at heart, whether on a small scale or a large, but their tendency is to crumble when faced by any sort of opposition. A miserable ram emerges in such circumstances; and when bruised, bleeding or defeated Arietians are at their most vulnerable and liable to compensate by over-indulging. Providing this is recognised and accepted as being the case, then members of this sign are half way to beating their obesity.

When down, the Arietian needs to be encouraged into hatching a new scheme. If the lost enthusiasm can somehow be re-ignited, it will oust the new-found bad habit, and the Arietian will go out once more prepared to do battle with the world. The Aries woman may find it more difficult to overcome overweight, for in general

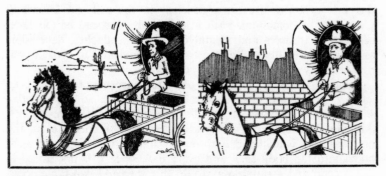

When his pioneering instincts are frustrated the Arietian eats to compensate

she takes her emotional life more seriously. When apathy sets in after a failed enterprise or an unsuccessful romance, she is often a pathetic sight. But in most cases the damage done during such a period rarely exceeds a few pounds, so ignore her when she says she's put on two stone—exaggeration is yet another characteristic of Aries. It may be true that her clothes are a size too small now, that a roll of fat is becoming quite visible around her midriff, but by no stretch of the imagination does she usually fit the description fat.

Life clearly needs to be restored to its proper perspective. Most of us possess a suit or dress that has always been too large, a bad purchase bought in a weak moment, and it is just that garment— or anything loose, flowing or that little bit too big—that the Arietian should extract from the wardrobe. For as soon as the Arietian can sit down with ease, eat a meal without finding it necessary to undo a button or a zip, he or she will begin to feel slimmer. At the same time that head must be kept busy and active with plans for the long-term future. Of course it isn't always as easy to put to rights one's emotional life; it's just not feasible to arange for Mr or Miss Right to arrive on the doorstep. But it's worth remembering that not all members of the opposite sex are attracted to the beanpole figure, and make the most of the new-found curves while they last.

WHAT KIND OF DIET?

If you're a health food fanatic, or simply interested in bio-chemistry, you may be interested to know that those born under the sign of Aries are often deficient in the cell salt known as phosphate of potassium. Such a lack in the diet can be the cause of nervous troubles and mental disorders, headaches, depression, and general debility and exhaustion (it is advisable to consult your doctor if any of these symptoms persist).

Some of the foods richest in phosphate are tomatoes, red beet, lemons, grapefruit, celery, parsnips and apples, so the Arietian should ensure that his or her diet regularly includes these foods. Arietian types must constantly keep their flow of energy even, and one way this is achieved is through Vitamin B. This needs to be taken into the body each and every day, since it is not stored in the system, and a simple way to do this is to add two tablespoons of brewers' yeast with celery flavouring to your gravies, stews, broths and meat loaves. Alternatively, sprinkle a tablespoonful of wheatgerm over your hot and cold cereals which is a delicous way to add B vitamins. Wheatgerm can also be used to coat food, in place of breadcrumbs, and to make gravies richer; put a few spoonfuls in whatever you bake, including waffles or pancakes.

Bearing in mind the fact that Arietians tend to bore easily, so that sticking to the diet can have its difficulties, it is suggested that after adhering to the following diets for a couple of weeks the Arietian extracts a day from one of the other eleven signs in order to provide a little variety. Monotony is the easiest way to discourage those trying to lose weight. As Aries is ruled by Mars, a planet shared by subject Scorpio, it is to the latter's diet sheet that Arietians can refer for revitalisation of their diet.

THE SEVEN-DAY ARIETIAN DIET

Monday

Breakfast: ½ grapefruit
1 boiled egg
1 slice wholemeal or rye bread
1 cup tea or coffee, with 1 tablespoon milk, no sugar

Lunch: Medium portion (4 oz) lamb's liver, fried in little oil
½ cup brussels sprouts
½ cup carrots
½ cup skimmed milk

Dinner: 4 tablespoonfuls cottage cheese on bed of lettuce
¼ medium-sized cucumber, sliced
1 fresh apple
½ cup skimmed milk

Tuesday

Breakfast: ½ cup strawberries
1 scrambled egg on wholemeal or rye bread (no butter)
1 cup tea or coffee, with 1 tablespoon milk, no sugar

Lunch: 1 thin slice of lean ham
½ cup canned peas
½ cup plums or cherries
½ cup skimmed milk

Dinner: 2 boiled eggs
1 large sliced tomato
1 stick celery
small portion of watermelon
½ cup skimmed milk

Wednesday

Breakfast: Small bowl of cereal with about 6 strawberries or raspberries
1 slice wholemeal or rye bread with 1 teaspoonful butter
½ cup skimmed milk

Lunch: 1 medium serving grilled lean fish, sprinkled with
                    lemon and parsley
                $\frac{1}{2}$ cup cauliflower or turnip greens
                $\frac{1}{2}$ cup blackberries or loganberries
                1 cup lemon tea, no sugar
Dinner: 1 medium slice corned beef
                1 tomato
                $\frac{1}{4}$ medium cucumber
                1 stick celery
                $\frac{1}{2}$ cup skimmed milk

Thursday

Breakfast: 1 poached egg on 1 slice wholemeal or rye toast
                    (no butter)
                1 cup lemon tea or black coffee
Lunch: Medium portion liver (beef or lamb)
                $\frac{1}{2}$ cup cauliflower or broccoli
                $\frac{1}{2}$ cup rhubarb or plums
                $\frac{1}{2}$ cup skimmed milk
Dinner: 1 medium-sized potato baked in jacket
                $\frac{1}{2}$ tablespoonful butter
                3 tablespoonfuls cottage cheese
                1 grated raw carrot
                1 medium-sized fresh peach
                $\frac{1}{2}$ cup skimmed milk

Friday

Breakfast: $\frac{1}{2}$ cup tinned grapefruit
                1 scrambled egg on rye bread (no butter)
                1 cup tea or coffee, with 1 tablespoon milk, no sugar
Lunch: 1 medium portion lean veal or lamb
                $\frac{1}{2}$ cup cabbage or Brussels sprouts
                $\frac{1}{2}$ cup cherries or loganberries
                $\frac{1}{2}$ cup skimmed milk
Dinner: 2 hard-boiled eggs
                3 tablespoonfuls cottage cheese
                1 stick celery
                $\frac{1}{4}$ medium cucumber
                1 fresh pear or peach
                $\frac{1}{2}$ cup skimmed milk

Saturday

Breakfast: 1 small bowl cereal sprinkled with tablespoonful of
                brewers' yeast
                ½ cup skimmed milk
Lunch: 2 lamb kidneys
                ½ cup cauliflower or spinach
                ½ cup spring greens
                1 cup black coffee or lemon tea, no sugar
Dinner: 1 medium portion fish sprinkled with parsley or
                lemon juice
                ½ cup aubergine slices or 5 sticks asparagus
                1 apple or 4 oz grapes
                1 cup skimmed milk

Sunday

Breakfast: ½ cup stewed apple or ½ grapefruit
                1 boiled egg with 1 slice wholemeal bread and 1
                teaspoonful butter
                ½ cup skimmed milk, or 1 cup tea or coffee with 1
                tablespoonful milk, no sugar
Lunch: 1 jacket potato with medium portion lean meat or
                fish
                1 large tomato, sliced
                a few lettuce leaves sprayed with lemon juice
                1 cup lime or lemon juice
Dinner: 2 lamb kidneys or small portion liver
                ½ cup carrots and mushrooms
                ½ cup apricots or blackberries
                1 cup skimmed milk

EXOTIC ARIETIAN RECIPE

Aries rules England, Denmark, Germany and Poland, and Arietians will find that food from these countries is particularly
appealing. Therefore when you have finished your diet why not
treat yourself to the German dish below? (A hint for seducers:
this dish is sure to increase your chances if you are trying to turn
on a Ram!)

Gefullte Hammelbrust (Stuffed Breast of Lamb)

3 lb breast of lamb	red wine or sour cream
¾ lb mushrooms	flour
1 large onion	

Bone the lamb and stuff with a mixture of chopped mushrooms and onions. Sprinkle with salt and pepper, roll and tie it with string or secure it with skewers. Rub the outside with melted butter, place in a baking tin, and when meat begins to brown baste with boiling water or stock. When meat is tender, take it from the pan and thicken the gravy. Add either red wine or sour cream to flavour. Serve the meat and sauce separately.

HOW DO YOU SHAPE UP AS AN ARIETIAN?

1. Do you have more than your fair share of headaches and neuralgia?
2. Do you frequently grab a quick sandwich or alcoholic drink instead of lunch?
3. Do you drink more than 8 cups of tea or coffee in one day?
4. Do you prefer to watch sport rather than participate?
5. Do you do your shopping in the closest shops so that you won't have far to walk?
6. Do you prefer to drive to work?
7. Are you out of breath when you climb more than 30 steps?
8. Does your partner complain of a lack of interest in things sexual?

If you answer "Yes" to more than 3 of the above then it's likely that you are an Arietian not only heading for overweight but also health problems. (And I bet you're an old crosspatch!)

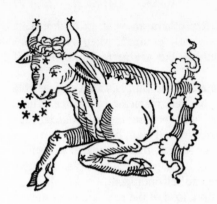

Taurus (the bull)

The sign of the builder or producer

April 21—May 21

The first earth sign: Stubborn, steadfast, systematic, kind-hearted, persevering, musical

Ruler: Venus   **Gems:** Moss-agate, emerald

Colours: Blue, pink   **Metal:** Copper

GENERAL CHARACTERISTICS

Taureans are not as mentally active as their Arietian friends but have a strong fund of good common sense. Neither idealists nor dreamers they are cautious, constructive and stable. Their motto is "one foot after another" until the goal is reached. They are industrious, patient and practical, but conservative first and foremost and like to identify with the traditional, the tried and the true. Once they have made up their minds they stick quite stubbornly to a course of action. They're not afraid of hard work; in fact they are dedicated to it, and obstacles only make them more persistent. They have untold reserves of energy and are capable of waiting a long time for their plans to mature. Sometimes they are overly tenacious; when an appeal has been made to their feelings they can stick to a losing cause long after others know it to be hopeless. They become obstinate, even violently enraged, when anyone tries to drive them into doing something, but are perfectly amenable if approached in the right way.

When it comes to financial dealings the Bull is sound and reliable and would make an excellent banker, manager or trustee. Those born under this sign are careful with their savings and assets; they like both money and the possessions it can buy. They have an innate sense of beauty but prefer objects that are useful as well as beautiful. In contrast to the well-integrated Taureans, negative types can be lazy, luxury-loving and self-indulgent.

Venus endows its subjects with a love of the arts and of romance; a Taurean may not have a silver tongue or look particularly sensitive, but when you get to know him he has a large heart. Losing his temper, he is slow to rise and slow to fall, so don't expect a flash-in-the-pan argument.

The Taurean woman makes an excellent mate and shines as a hostess. Like her brother she has a morbid fear of debt, and keeps a strict eye on her comforts and needs. She really prefers to be dominated by her man, and can help considerably in furthering his ambitions; but if she loses confidence in or respect for him she's quite capable of taking the reins herself and organising both their lives realistically.

Taurus is an excellent sign to belong to, unless you are of the weaker variety. Then excess vitality is bottled up instead of flowing out freely to help others. These types are essentially self-centred and quite incapable of seeing anyone else's point of view, and the normally splendid persistence shows itself as unbelievable obstinacy and pig-headedness.

Famous Taureans: Perry Como, Bing Crosby, Salvador Dali, Moshe Dayan, Queen Elizabeth II, Duke Ellington, Ella Fitzgerald, Henry Fonda, Hirohito, Karl Marx, Robespierre, Bertrand Russell, Shakespeare, Benjamin Spock, Barbra Streisand, Shirley Temple, Orson Welles.

LOVE, SEX AND THE TAUREAN

Physical attraction is very important to Taureans and Platonic love does not exist for them. They are natural and direct in any close relationship. Indeed, in his anxiety to know exactly where he stands a Bull will pursue until accepted or rejected. The instincts are such that the Taurean has absolutely no sense of shame.

This type is often a late developer physically, but nevertheless attracts admirers from an early age. He or she rarely falls in love until the right person arrives on the scene, and once this happens Taureans are tenacious but also tremendously affectionate and demonstrative. They love to give and receive gifts, sweet messages and flowers—all the conventional accoutrements of love. The Taurean disposition is kindly and cheerful, which makes for popularity. The home is greatly appreciated and Taureans ensure that one way or another they can afford the comforts and luxuries of life, for they intend to spend much of their time within the home.

Sexually Taureans are normally straightforward and, while there is nothing wrong with this, it is all too easy for boredom to creep into their relationships. Ideally the Taurean should at least try to experiment a little and not worry about becoming perverted. There's no point in any member of the opposite sex attempting to force this type into different behaviour; patience and subtlety are called for.

FASHION AND THE TAUREAN

Taurus subjects are endowed with excellent taste which needs to be particularly observed when those extra pounds of fat have been allowed to gather. This type is often attracted to lighter shades but clearly this is ill-advised as it does little to disguise those unwanted bulges. Taureans are fond of jewellery, particularly necklaces, but it is recommended that this be kept to a minimum during the attempt to recapture that sylphlike silhouette. Those of this sign usually possess a keen sense of touch and smell, so splash out on some expensive perfume to make you feel great. And there's nothing to stop you being totally outrageous when it comes to underwear; the Taurus woman gets a delicious thrill from knowing that while she may look demure and plain on the outside underneath she's feeling daringly wicked (satins are particularly recommended—the very touch of them is enough to boost even the most deflated Taurean ego). It might not be a bad idea for the overweight Taurean woman to bear in mind that many men prefer larger women, who can look far sexier in the nude than their skinnier sisters; she should make the most of her ample breasts with low necklines and the appropriate bra. This will appeal to the exhibitionist lurking within most women, will put her in greater demand and will help to sustain her when life becomes depressing due to the lack of those sticky cream buns.

PHYSICAL CHARACTERISTICS AND HEALTH

The Taurean man tends to have a large frame, often overweight; a square-shaped head with thick, fine hair; dark eyes; a full lower lip; a thick neck and sloping shoulders.

The Taurean woman tends to have a large body, with a good bust and bulky hips; well marked eyebrows, which give a determined expression; a fleshy nose, and sensuous mouth; sloping shoulders.

Taurus rules the throat, neck, ears and jaws, the base of the brain and also the heart. All Taureans possess great physical endurance, though once they have come down with a disease they may be slow to recuperate. Laryngitis is a fairly common Taurean disorder, and money problems often undermine their health. Fortunately, however, the Bull is normally an extremely strong animal, and those born under this sign are likely to accept life more calmly and take better care of themselves than, say, Arietians or Geminians.

CAUSES OF TAUREAN OBESITY AND HOW TO COPE

This is the sign of the gourmand and the epicurean and regrettably it seems to account for more overweight people than any other. It doesn't take much to send the bull on a food binge, for it's hard for Taureans to deny themselves pleasures connected with the throat. All born under this sign feel they must eat, drink and make love to excess. When denied the latter they rely on the former. This is an unfortunate habit and the accompanying complexes produce an array of inhibitions. It's a common vicious circle: Taureans eat to compensate for sexual frustration, but the fatter they become the harder they imagine it will be to fulfil this sexual appetite.

Apart from this, Taureans have problems with their famous stubbornness which in many instances makes it almost impossible for them to admit that they are overweight at all. It's a good idea for the Taurean to take a long, cold look in the bedroom mirror and try to be honest about the image that greets him or her.

The members of this sign are almost proud of their giant capacity (which may seem like greed to other people) and over the years their stomach grows so accustomed to being subjected to vast amounts of food that it stretches, and when suddenly starved in the form of a diet it cries out in loud protest. The Taurean's admitted liking for food turns into something of a love affair when he or she has financial or emotional difficulties. Fortunately our bull-like friend does possess splendid determination and when this characteristic has a chance to exercise itself the results can be startling. But the first step towards acquiring that much-desired slimness is a straightforward look at the reflection in the mirror.

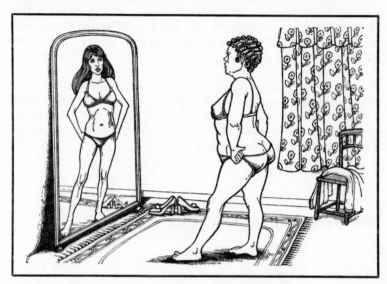

There's no hope for a Taurean who can't face the facts

WHAT KIND OF DIET?

Interestingly enough, Taureans are frequently deficient in the cell salt commonly known as sulphate of soda, and where this deficiency occurs there is a tendency to disorders of the liver, kidneys and pancreas. This can lead to troubles such as jaundice, diabetes, asthma, rheumatism, enlarged prostate and constipation. The sodium in the body controls the correct distribution of calcium. Some of the foods richest in sodium are celery, apples, spinach, radishes, lettuce, strawberries, pomegranate; the Taurean can never really eat too much of these foods and should try to consciously include them in his or her diet (the lazier way of obtaining the required natrium sulphuricum is in tablet form, from a reputable chemist). Taureans may be healthiest on a near-vegetarian diet.

As Taurus is ruled by Venus, a planet shared by Libra, it is to the Libran menus that Taureans can refer when they wish to revitalise their diet, or simply when they need a change.

SPECIAL TAUREAN RECIPES

The following two recipes are not necessarily to be included in a slimming diet but are meant specifically to be taken as a tonic when the Taurean is feeling down.

Taurean Fruit Salad
Mash a few fresh strawberries and add a finely grated apple. Mix the two together, adding a few well ground nuts. Spread this mixture on buttered wholemeal bread.

Taurean Savoury Salad
Chop up some young and tender spinach leaves fairly finely. Mix a little fresh cream with a small portion of honey and a few drops of orange or lemon juice. Mix this with the spinach, then arrange it on the leaves of a young crisp lettuce.

THE SEVEN-DAY TAUREAN DIET

Monday

Breakfast: ½ grapefruit or 10 strawberries
                  black coffee
Mid-morning: 1 glass buttermilk or tomato juice
Lunch: 2 hard-boiled eggs with 1 slice wholemeal bread
                  chopped carrot salad
                  1 glass lemonade
Mid-afternoon: 1 cup lemon tea
Dinner: 1 cup clear soup
                  2 slices lean beef or lamb
                  combination salad of cucumber, radish, celery
                  black coffee
Before retiring: A good time each day to take vitamins, or 1 table-
                  spoon brewers' yeast in glass of fruit or vegetable
                  juice, or yogurt

Tuesday

Breakfast: 1 slice orange or medium baked apple
                  black coffee
Mid-morning: 1 glass yogurt or 1 cup hot broth

Lunch:	1 large hamburger with chopped parsley and onion
	½ head of lettuce sprinkled with lemon juice and vegetable salt
	1 cup lemon tea
Mid-afternoon:	1 cup clear soup
Dinner:	1 large slice lean roast beef or 2 large slices roast chicken
	carrot and celery sticks
	½ cup spinach
	1 grilled grapefruit

Wednesday

Breakfast:	1 baked apple or apple sauce
	black coffee
Mid-morning:	1 glass buttermilk or 1 cup hot broth
Lunch:	2 eggs boiled or poached, topped with ½ cup stewed tomatoes
	chopped carrot and apple salad
	1 cup tea or coffee, no sugar
Mid-afternoon:	1 glass lemonade or 1 cup clear soup
Dinner:	Fresh Taurean Fruit Salad
	2 grilled lean lamb chops
	½ cup green peas sprinkled with parsley
	black coffee

Thursday

Breakfast:	½ orange or ½ grapefruit
	black coffee
Mid-morning:	1 glass yogurt or tomato juice
Lunch:	2 slices grilled liver
	chopped cabbage and green pepper salad
	1 cup tea or coffee, no sugar
Mid-afternoon:	1 cup lemon tea or 1 glass lemonade
Dinner:	Vegetable juice cocktail
	1 large veal chop with fresh celery
	½ pomegranate

Friday

Breakfast:	Fruit or tomato juice
	black coffee

Mid-morning: 1 glass buttermilk or yogurt
Lunch: 2 scrambled eggs with chopped spinach/2 poached
                   eggs on 1 slice toast
                celery or carrot sticks
                1 cup tea or coffee, no sugar
Mid-afternoon: 1 cup lemon tea or 1 cup clear soup
Dinner: 1 glass grapefruit juice
                1 large slice grilled sole, white fish or halibut
                ½ cup stewed tomatoes and celery
                ½ tin mandarin oranges or ½ grapefruit

Saturday

Breakfast: ½ cup strawberries or 1 sliced orange
                black coffee
Mid-morning: 1 glass buttermilk, yogurt or tomato juice
Lunch: 3 tablespoons cottage cheese with chives or onions
                   on a bed of lettuce
                raw celery and carrots
                1 cup lemon tea
Dinner: 1 grilled grapefruit
                2 slices roast lamb
                ½ cup spinach/green beans/broccoli/brussels sprouts
                baked apple
                1 cup coffee, no sugar

Sunday

Breakfast: 2 scrambled eggs on 1 slice wholewheat toast
                1 glass buttermilk, yogurt or tomato juice
Lunch: Taurean Savoury Salad mixed with ½ cup cold meat
                baked apple or apple sauce
                1 cup lemon tea or 1 glass lemonade
Dinner: 1 cup clear soup
                ½ grilled chicken
                ½ cup cauliflower or spinach
                4 or 5 stewed apricots
                1 cup coffee, no sugar

EXOTIC TAUREAN RECIPES

Taurus rules Ireland, Switzerland, Persia and Cyprus and food from these countries has particular appeal for Taureans. Therefore when you have finished your diet you may like to treat yourself to the Swiss or the Irish dish below. (Hint for seducers: either of these dishes is bound to increase your chances with a stubborn Bull.)

Zurich Ratsherrentopf

1 teacup potatoes, cubed	$\frac{1}{2}$ teacup diced larding bacon
$\frac{1}{2}$ teacup butter	$\frac{1}{2}$ teacup mushrooms
$\frac{1}{4}$ lb (110 grams) fillet of pork	$1\frac{1}{2}$ teacups peas, boiled
$\frac{1}{4}$ lb fillet of veal	2 tomatoes, grilled
$\frac{1}{4}$ lb fillet of beef	

Roast potatoes in 4 tablespoons butter in a 350°F oven (gas mark 4) for 30 minutes. Meanwhile sauté pork, veal and beef in 3 tablespoons butter; set aside and keep warm. Mix larding bacon and mushrooms with 1 tablespoon melted butter and mix with potatoes. Return to oven for 5 minutes.

Arrange potatoes on one side of serving platter and the peas on the other. Place the meat on the potatoes and the tomatoes on the peas.

Serves 2.

Veal "Collar of Gold"

4 tablespoons butter	5 teacups cream
4 slices veal, pounded thin	salt
$\frac{1}{2}$ teacup sliced button mushrooms	pepper
4 tablespoons chopped onions	1 tablespoon chopped parsley
2 teacups sherry	

Clarify butter in frying pan. Add veal; brown and set aside. Sauté mushrooms and onion in the same pan. Add sherry and cream. Reduce sauce until it is of medium thickness. Season with salt and pepper. Return veal to pan, sprinkle with chopped parsley, and serve.

Serves 4.

Wine suggestion: claret.

HOW DO YOU SHAPE UP AS A TAUREAN?

1. Do you suffer from aching neck muscles?
2. Are you a quick eater? (No extra points for sparks made with knife and fork!)
3. Have you refused your partner sexually more than once this week?
4. Have you fallen asleep in front of the television more than twice this week?
5. Do you like to watch the garden growing, but don't know a dibber from a trowel?
6. Do you have a weakness for potatoes?
7. Can you eat more than most other people at one sitting?
8. Do you know your own weight?

If you answer "Yes" to more than 3 of the above questions then you're probably on your way to being an overweight Taurean with health problems (and you could be something of an irritable Bullock).

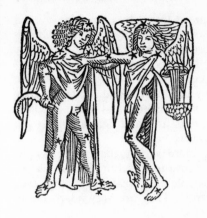

Gemini (the twins)

The sign of the artist or inventor

May 22—June 21

The first air sign: Restless, versatile, clever, exuberant, expressive,
expressive, artistic, talkative
Ruler: Mercury **Gems:** Beryl, aquamarine
Colour: Yellow **Metal:** Quicksilver

GENERAL CHARACTERISTICS

Gemini is the most versatile sign, and Geminians are intellectual
and many-sided. They have sensitive, highly-strung dispositions,
fine minds and good memories; but, unless there are other indications in the birth chart, they are not particularly original. Nevertheless, they are very intuitive and receptive to knowledge. They are
capable of expressing in speech or writing a continuous stream of
ideas, for they are logical and adept in argument.

Geminians are never so happy as when they are leading a double
life. They are likely to have dual professions, and two or more
romantic interests at once. They may have several hobbies or other ·
spare time diversions. In the more negative types, this bent can

degenerate into a tendency to spread themselves too thin, doing a lot of things haphazardly and nothing specially well. These types fritter their time away, not concentrating their energies sufficiently to achieve excellence or success; they become destructive and restless, unable to stick to any occupation for long. The positive Geminian types, however, display much force and initiative. They are definite in their views, have many talents and make excellent management executives. They are as firm and dependable as the negative types are irresolute and irresponsible.

Ordinarily Geminians require more variety than other people. They need frequent vacations and love to travel to different places. If there are changes in their schedule and breaks in routine, they tend to work much more efficiently. They are very adaptable to people, situations and environments.

The male Geminian in particular has a desire to influence those around him, which makes it impossible for him to suffer alone or in silence. He loves to make friends, and when they misunderstand him his suffering often seems like martyrdom. Exultation accompanying any achievement is generally followed by critical inspection (for he is the most introspective of men) and a circling round in the vain hope that he may eventually come to know himself.

The Geminian woman needs plenty of activity about her, and she usually manages to find it or create it. Nine times out of ten, tantrum-throwing is her way of keeping everyone on their mental toes. Men are attracted to her stimulating company, though trying to hold her interest can prove quite a challenge; she is always out for something to discuss or criticise. Don't be thrown if, in the middle of a world-shattering debate, she decides that your hair is parted on the wrong side. She has a tendency to gossip and this can lead to tense situations. But for the most part the Geminian is charming and fun to anyone who enjoys a surprise element in their lives.

Famous Geminians: Tony Curtis, Bob Dylan, Sir Anthony Eden, Judy Garland, George V, Bob Hope, John F. Kennedy, Christopher Lee, Paul McCartney, Marilyn Monroe, Laurence Olivier, Rosalind Russell, Tito, Queen Victoria, John Wayne.

LOVE, SEX AND THE GEMINIAN

Geminians may put up with domesticity but are not likely to participate wholeheartedly in family life. They are ruled by their minds, so their emotions can be somewhat shallow, leading to a superficial attitude to relationships. People born under this sign rarely like to be touched or fondled, and become claustrophobic rather quickly. They tend to have mental and ideal attractions rather than physical ones. They also have a tendency to flirt; their interest is easily roused but they have a short attention span. They don't really want concrete attachments and while they enjoy being with someone who catches their fancy they would be abashed to be taken seriously. They're basically intellectual about love: they like to read about it and think about it; they seldom feel it. Their admirers for the most part come in pairs or large numbers—if the Gemini man could keep a harem and the Gemini woman its male equivalent, these two would indeed be happy.

Most Geminians learn young to rely heavily on sexual fantasy, and it is common for this type to want to indulge in elaborate games which stimulate the over-active mental faculties and allow the assumption of any role appropriate to the mood. But inhibition may prevent the Geminian from openly acknowledging these needs, or it may not be easy to find a willing and imaginative partner. Light pornography may set things in motion—the written word rather than explicit pictures. Novelty, challenge and excitement are the essential three ingredients in the Geminian love life, and without them frustration results. With regard to sexual appetite, Geminians are extremists. When involved with someone who works to make lovemaking an art, they can be insatiable, spurred on by willingness to learn. However, coupled with a partner who is unable to come up with the odd surprise, then the Geminian sexual appetite will fade. This can happen so subtly that the subject may be totally unaware of it until it is brought to his or her attention.

FASHION AND THE GEMINIAN

This is an ultra-elegant sign, for normally those born under it are tall, slim and naturally poised—those enviable types who not only do justice to Balmain but who can also look suitably groomed wrapped in an old blanket. Such characters are inclined to take their appearance for granted. It's only when those extra inches creep round the waistline that they suddenly realise they don't look quite so well dressed as they used to. Where once they were able to slop around the house in an old shirt and jeans and still look sexy, overweight Geminians find that the casual appeal is gone and they look like an unmade bed. It may be a while before this fact sinks in. This is the type who up till now has been able to follow any fashion, no matter how extreme; but that cute little blonde who used to trip along in her platform shoes looks pretty ridiculous when she puts on another couple of stone.

How to adjust to the new situation? Well, having faced facts the dieting Geminian must make a few changes to his or her wardrobe. Anything too figure-hugging or young and trendy should be temporarily forgotten. Most of all, those bright, garish patterns that attract Geminians are definitely out; they are possibly the worst designs to wear when you are a little overweight. If such an individual insists on wearing such an outfit he or she will only end up feeling like Moby Dick. Pick out the looser garments; there's no need to wear widow's weeds but at least choose softer, plain colours. It won't be long before you're back to your usual sleek self. Remember, too, that Gemini rules the arms and that while your body may grow a bit lumpy those lithe limbs of yours rarely succumb to fat; so during the warmer weather why not stock up on flattering sleeveless tops.

PHYSICAL CHARACTERISTICS AND HEALTH

The Geminian man tends to have a lean body with long, slender limbs; light silky hair; an animated face with wide-apart eyes, and a wide, expressive mouth.

The Geminian woman tends to have a slim, sometimes thin, body with a small bust; high cheekbones; a wide mouth; light, twinkling eyes; a pale skin which tans easily.

Subjects of this sign tend to be clever with their hands and like to use them constantly, for Gemini rules the hands, arms and shoulders, as well as the upper respiratory system, the nerves and that part of the brain controlling higher thought processes. The health of Geminians is not robust and there is a danger of lung complaints if care is not taken. Many born under this sign are chain smokers which is obviously a danger to the health. Colds are often contracted easily, especially when the Geminian is down. Nervous energy can carry subjects of this sign through most things but deserts them the moment a task becomes dull. Nervous exhaustion frequently follows their tremendous outbursts, and health needs to be treated in much the same way as a child's with, above all, plenty of fresh air, sleep and sensible diet. Once the Geminian recognises this he or she will benefit immensely, but a degree of rebellion may be displayed against this advice due to Geminian immaturity. This type takes a little longer to grow up than most, and some never quite make it.

CAUSES OF GEMINIAN OBESITY AND HOW TO COPE

Fortunately, most members of this sign, the least food-conscious, manage to retain their sylphlike figures into advanced years; their nervous energy simply burns up excess calories. There are, of course, exceptions and a plump Geminian completely contradicts the old idea that fat people are jolly, being more often than not irritable and bad-tempered. Boredom is generally the reason this

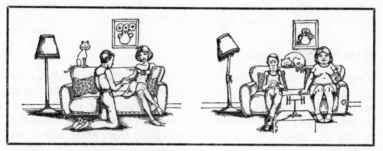

The Geminian eats when bored

character finds it necessary to indulge the appetite to excess. Those of this sign need constant mental stimulation and when this is not forthcoming they are a miserable sight. If subjected to routine and uninteresting work, or a dreary partner, some Geminians will eat just for the sake of keeping occupied.

Having established that the Geminian's own particular devil that causes those inches to accumulate is an over-active head, we know that the cure is to keep it busy. If the Geminian is not inclined to study or produce literary masterpieces then such energy is directed into the love life. The Geminian is a true Don Juan, preferring to run at least a dozen members of the opposite sex at once, and just keeping up with the dramas that this entails is enough to keep him mentally active and therefore slim. So it is our married subject who is likely to gather the pounds—and regrettably Geminians all too often rush into marriage. This is unwise mainly because not only must there be physical compatibility in a mate but, more important, intellectual rapport too. Without it, once the initial glow has worn off the relationship the Geminian will be bored out of his or her head. New interests and challenges are the ways to combat such a state of affairs. The worst thing a Geminian can do is to sink into a state of apathy, curl up in front of the television and switch off the outside world, and those who do are the few fat members of this sign. Geminians are not very good at gauging their weight, so check with the tables at the front of the book. The Geminian urge to concoct their own cures for everything can be disastrous. Drug abuse is frequently found with this sign. It cannot be stressed too strongly that drugs should never be taken for slimming, because (1) they are habit-forming; (2) eventually they have a destructive effect on the Geminian's delicate nervous system; (3) they usually have some side-effects; and (4) once they are discontinued the fat often starts to accumulate at a faster rate than before. Sensible dieting, then, is the only way out.

WHAT KIND OF DIET?

Those born under the sign of Gemini are often deficient in the cell salt known as potassium chloride, and such a deficiency may result in a tendency towards inflammations, catarrh, a sluggish liver, swollen glands, swellings and congestions. The following foods rich in this salt should be included in the daily diet: green beans, turnips, cheese, goat's milk, brussels sprouts, cauliflower, lettuce, watercress, pineapple. Also very important where Geminians are concerned is Vitamin D, which not only helps give us healthy bones and hard white teeth but in addition helps to keep the nerves relaxed; yet few foods have enough of this vitamin to supply our daily needs, so it is a good idea to use milk and other foods enriched with this vitamin, especially during the winter months. It can also be taken in the form of cod liver oil capsules. Another source of this vitamin given to us by nature is the sun, and because orange lemon and grapefruit peels have been exposed to the sun they all contain Vitamin D. So use grated citrus peel wherever possible in baking or other cooking; for example, it is delicious in stewed dried fruits.

As Gemini is ruled by Mercury, the planet shared by subjects of Virgo, it is to the latter's diet sheet that the Geminian should refer when variety is needed. Included in this book is a special diet for those who want to put on weight and since Geminians are more prone to suffer from lack of inches than excess of them the skinnier subjects of this sign may find that section beneficial.

SPECIAL GEMINIAN RECIPES

The following are all rich in Vitamin D and, though not necessarily to be included in a slimming diet, are extremely good for the run-down Geminian.

Honey Butter
Warm some fresh unsalted butter until all water evaporates. Mix two parts of the butter to one part of honey and beat until it is of a creamy consistency. Spread on wholemeal bread.

Geminian Salad (can be used in diet)
Arrange crisp lettuce leaves in a salad bowl. Grate some raw turnip and carrot, slice tomatoes, and chop some spinach finely. Pile these neatly on to the lettuce, then sprinkle with a little grated cheese. Garnish with watercress.

Geminian Cocktail
Extract the juice from a fresh pineapple. Pulp a few strawberries and add them to the juice. Dilute with a little water. Keep the mixture cool until ready to serve it.

THE SEVEN-DAY GEMINIAN DIET

Monday

Breakfast: 1 large glass fruit juice
1 boiled egg with 1 slice rye bread, ½ oz butter
black coffee

Lunch: 4 oz sardines
1 chopped carrot and 1 large tomato
1 cup lemon tea or clear soup

Dinner: 2 slices lean lamb
Geminian Salad
1 cup coffee

Before retiring: A good time to take your recommended cod liver oil capsules; a tablespoonful of brewers' yeast in fruit juice is also extremely beneficial and should be taken every night of the diet.

Tuesday

Breakfast: 1 sliced orange
1 piece wholemeal bread with scraping of butter
1 cup tea or coffee, no sugar

Lunch: 4 oz halibut or mackerel with chopped parsley or onion
½ head of lettuce sprinkled with lemon juice
½ cup skimmed milk

Dinner: 1 medium portion lean liver
                   ½ cup spinach
                   carrots and celery sticks
                   black coffee

Wednesday

Breakfast: 1 glass Geminian Cocktail
                   1 egg yolk stirred into ½ cup milk
                   1 baked apple
Lunch: 1 poached or boiled egg, with ½ cup stewed tomatoes
                   1 large apple
                   1 cup tea or coffee, no sugar
Dinner: 2 grilled lean lamb chops
                   ½ cup spinach
                   ½ cup loganberries
                   1 cup tea or coffee, no sugar

Thursday

Breakfast: 1 cup stewed apple
                   small bowl cereal
                   black coffee, no sugar
Lunch: 4 oz salmon or mackerel
                   2 oz cucumber, or ½ cup cauliflower
                   ½ cup rhubarb
                   1 cup tea or coffee, no sugar
Dinner: 1 slice cheese on toast topped with poached egg
                   1 sliced tomato and chopped carrot
                   1 stick celery
                   1 cup skimmed milk

Friday

Breakfast: 1 large glass Geminian Cocktail
                   1 sliced tomato on 1 slice wholemeal toast
                   black coffee
Lunch: 2 slices grilled liver
                   ½ cup chopped cabbage
                   ½ cup green pepper salad
                   1 yogurt
                   1 cup lemon tea

Dinner: 1 veal chop with cauliflower and cheese salad
                  1 stick celery
                  small piece watermelon
                  ½ cup skimmed milk

Saturday

Breakfast: 1 glass tomato juice
                  ½ grapefruit or orange
                  1 cup tea or coffee, no sugar
Lunch: 1 jacket potato with grated cheese
                  1 grated carrot and stick of celery
                  1 glass fruit juice
Dinner: 1 cup light soup
                  1 large slice white fish (sole or halibut)
                  ½ cup stewed tomatoes and celery
                  ½ cup strawberries
                  black coffee

Sunday

Breakfast: 1 glass orange juice
                  1 poached egg on slice of wholemeal bread
                  1 cup tea or coffee, no sugar
Lunch: 2 grilled kidneys
                  ½ cup broccoli or spinach and ½ cup green beans
                  ½ cup blackberries/blueberries/raspberries
Dinner: 4 oz lean steak with 1 oz chopped onion
                  ½ cup cauliflower sprinkled with grated cheese
                  1 large peach
                  ½ cup skimmed milk

EXOTIC GEMINIAN RECIPE

Gemini rules the USA, Belgium, Sardinia and Wales, and it is food from these countries that is likely to be most to the Geminian taste. After you have finished your diet is a good time to treat yourself to the American hamburger dish below—these are hamburgers with a difference. (Hint to seducers: this is a recipe bound to assist in turning on your schizophrenic Gemini friend!)

Hamburgers with Pizzaiola Sauce

2 lb lean sirloin or rump steak
1 oz unsalted butter
salt and black pepper

Sauce:

2 onions	2 oz mushroom caps
2 cloves of garlic	14 or 16 oz tin of tomatoes
2 green peppers	2 level teaspoons oregano (or marjoram)
1 dessertspoon olive oil	chili sauce
salt	black pepper

Trim any fat from the steak, cut it into pieces and put through the mincer (coarse plate). Shape the mince into 6 or 8 rounds, about 1½ inches thick. Avoid overhandling as this makes them tough. Leave the hamburgers to rest while preparing the sauce.

Peel and mince the onions and garlic. Remove stalks and seeds from the peppers and cut them crossways into thin slices. Heat the oil in a deep, heavy-based frying pan and, over a gentle heat, cook onions and garlic until they are golden brown. Add pepper slices and continue cooking for 15 minutes. Wash or peel the mushrooms, chop them roughly and add to the pan together with the tomatoes and the oregano or marjoram. Cover and cook for another 10 minutes. Season to taste with chili sauce, salt and freshly ground black pepper. Leave pan over low heat while cooking the hamburgers.

Melt the butter in a heavy-based frying pan; for pink-rare hamburgers fry 4 minutes each side, for medium, add 2 minutes each side more. Sprinkle with salt and pepper.

Put hamburgers on a hot serving dish and pour the sauce over them.

HOW DO YOU SHAPE UP AS A GEMINIAN?

1. Do you suffer with aching shoulders?
2. Do you smoke more than 15 cigarettes a day?
3. Are you bored with your job?
4. Do you often walk about while eating or drinking?
5. Are sandwiches and cakes the only lunch you have time for?
6. Have you been with the same partner for more than 3 years?
7. Do you watch television more than 4 nights a week?
8. Do you always make love in the same position?

If you answer "Yes" to more than 3 of these questions then you're a Geminian heading for both weight and health problems—in fact you're probably something of a nervous wreck already.

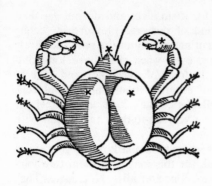

Cancer (the crab)
The sign of the prophet and teacher

June 22—July 22

The first water sign: Tenacious, patient, sensitive, sympathetic, changeable
Ruler: The Moon **Gems:** Moss-agate, emerald
Colour: Violet **Metal:** Silver

GENERAL CHARACTERISTICS

There is more difference between active and passive types in Cancer than in any other sign. The active type is strong-willed and very persistent. Natives of this water sign have as corrosive an effect on anything they set out to change or destroy as the milling waves that eat away an ocean cliff. These people are masterful and tireless in their approach to life. The passive type on the other hand is lackadaisical and idle, taking the line of least resistance, come what may. However he will cling tenaciously to what he already has.

Both types are the product of their environment and are much influenced by their early training; they are usually very attached to their home and mother. Cancerians have an easy-going disposition and are faithful in love, a combination that makes for happiness in marriage. However they are sensitive and can be deeply hurt by criticism; when they feel sorry for themselves and do not get their own way, they may take a kind of perverse pleasure in feeling martyred. They are extremely sentimental about the past and rarely discard old ties and friendships, even when they have long outgrown them. They are especially fond of anecdotes and love to reminisce. They like all kinds of antiques, books and art objects, and they can become avid collectors. They have a real feel for history, at the same time as being very up-to-date and *au fait* with everything modern and current.

Cancerians' interests are domestic—particularly what goes on in the kitchen (often their downfall, for this may give them unwholesome appetites). They enjoy television, and also the theatre. They love to act and to receive publicity, and no audience is ever too small. Cancerians love fame and recognition, and this means their ambitions could take on an unusual form and the desire for power could lead to a high position from which they cannot be dislodged. It is rare indeed to see a Cancerian subject deposed once he or she has reached the heights of success.

The female of the species has all the vices and virtues of her brother crab; like him, she isn't as strong as other Sun signs, but her strength is the ability to love and cherish. A marked maternal instinct is to the fore of her personality. Unfortunately when this girl isn't able to find a true soul mate, it affects her far more deeply than it does those born under more resilient signs. When unhappy she can become a burden on friends and relatives, leaning heavily on their time and sympathies. The Cancerian woman is always at her best in the throes of matrimonial bliss. The right man doesn't have to be a millionaire, either. She will only feel inclined to spend, spend, spend if seeking an embrocation for sprained emotions. Buying her solid gold bracelets will obviously please her, but if she says "You shouldn't have", you can bet your bottom dollar that is exactly what she means.

Famous Cancerians: Yul Brynner, Pearl Buck, Marc Chagall, Erle Stanley Gardner, Edward Heath, Nelson Rockefeller, Richard Rodgers, Jane Russell, Jean-Paul Sartre.

LOVE, SEX AND THE CANCERIAN

Cancerian affections are generally deep and constant. Family ties and friendships are not weakened by time or distance, and in particular the bond between father and son is jealously guarded for it is close and often a source of inspiration. An emotional outlet is a prime requirement for the Cancerian's health and well-being. Rather than actually go out looking for love, they wait until it comes to them, and when pursued by the opposite sex they accept attentions gratefully, finding it difficult to resist advances. Cancerians are intensely and quietly sentimental and although they tend to take love very seriously they are apt to get over disappointment quickly despite what they will tell you. They are basically good humoured and therefore popular. They like their comforts and usually manage to acquire them. Cancerians have a natural tendency towards clannish activities and try to avoid being alone whenever possible. They seek the approval of others and so a fear of ridicule brings out the conventional side to the character as the Cancerian tries to avoid eccentricity.

This type may have read at some time articles which suggest that he or she is undersexed, but these should be dismissed. It is true that rarely are Cancerians consumed by lustful feelings; they are such complex characters and inclined towards self-pity and martyrdom—even masochism occasionally—that their baser instincts may remain dormant and suppressed, lest they be thought kinky or perverted. For the most part, Cancer is a romantic, gentle sign so it's very easy to take its subject for granted. Sexually speaking Cancerians need a lot of understanding. The Cancerian woman relates her sexuality to the man in her life and has at least to pretend to be in love before closing the bedroom door behind her. If that man refuses to understand this then there will be trouble. Her big watery eyes may hold the look of love but as soon as the other side of the bed has gone cold so will her pretence. It has to be romance, moonlight and love all the way for this type.

FASHION AND THE CANCERIAN

Few members of this sign manage to attain prominence on the world's best-dressed lists; Cancerians go for what delights the eye rather than what flatters the figure. Frequently they compensate for lack of flamboyance in the character by affecting the most way-out dress. And the more overweight the Cancerian is, the more unhappy he or she is, the more he or she tries to attract the limelight somehow—anyhow. That woman with the ludicrous hat sitting opposite you in the train, you don't think she actually believes she looks elegant, do you? Of course not—but at least you noticed her, and that was the object of the exercise.

False economy is another reason why Cancerians can hardly be accused of being overly smart. They are the proverbial bargain hunters. Open a Cancerian's wardrobe and you will discover two dozen pairs of cheap shoes, a score of nondescript dresses or suits that were such a snip they couldn't be resisted—invariably all items the rest of us wouldn't be seen dead in. The Cancerian would be well advised to curb the bargain-hunter within and put the money thus saved towards an outfit of real quality and one that above all is the correct size. You may have been a size 12 in your twenties but, let's face it, though you may still be able to squeeze yourself into the same dress, how many times has the zip been repaired? Stand sideways in front of the mirror and you'll see what I mean. Be honest about your measurements, if only to yourself. Buy a pair of trousers that fits you and allows you to breathe occasionally. Put those frills and bows away until your figure can do justice to them. A sensible attitude to your wardrobe and a careful selection of garments can do wonders for your figure before you lose so much as an inch. This may be the sign of the Crab, but do you really want to look like one?

PHYSICAL CHARACTERISTICS AND HEALTH

The Cancerian man usually has a medium build, with large hands and feet; a large skull with an overhanging brow and a pronounced lower jaw; a turned-up nose.

The Cancerian woman tends to have a long body with a good bust and large hips and thighs; large feet; a strong jaw; possibly short-sighted or deepset eyes; a pale skin.

Cancer rules the stomach, the breasts and the lower lungs. Cancerians love rich food and are inclined to eat much too quickly and troubles such as indigestion, ulcers and all digestive disorders can be expected. Obviously such complaints cannot be avoided without the right diet; worry also aggravates the situation, and this in turn can lead to defective circulation. A tendency to always fear the worst does not help members of this sign either. This is the sign of the hypochondriac—as those around any Cancerian will no doubt have realised—so it's difficult to know when the symptoms are genuine. The Cancerian imagination is such that psychosomatic illnesses are very easily generated. He or she may feel depressed or unloved and in an effort to gain attention may fabricate, for example, a touch of 'flu; and sure enough, by the end of the day the Cancerian is sniffing and snuffling with the best of them. If the morbid fantasies can be kept under control then Cancer is as strong a sign as any other. Cancerians frequently live to a ripe old age—

but try to get them to admit they're 100 per cent healthy and you'll have a difficult job on your hands.

CAUSES OF CANCERIAN OBESITY AND HOW TO COPE

Most Cancerians experience a weight problem at some point in their life, for when their sensitivity is at all upset they are inclined to lose complete self-control. Give this type a reason to feel unwanted and the martyr lurking within surfaces and goes on an orgy of

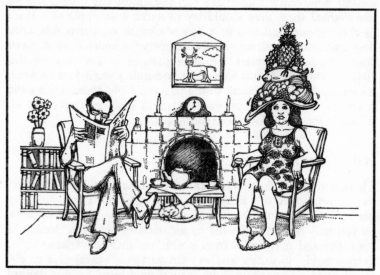

The Cancerian need for attention takes bizarre forms, and when unsuccessful what is left? Food!

overeating—often a desperate attempt to attract the notice of loved ones. Members of this sign may be greedy in a sly way, resorting to surreptitious snacks. Unfortunately this type is also the possessor of a sweet tooth; pounds of candy, biscuits and even evil sticky buns may be unconsciously consumed. Cancerians may be over-fond of alcohol, too, particularly gin, vodka and white wine. The wrong food leads to excess fat, and this is why Cancer is one of the heavier signs in the zodiac.

Furthermore, many born at this time refuse to face the fact that they are overweight, sporting clothes made for people three sizes smaller. It is the Cancerian mother who says of her chubby child, "It's only puppy fat," or "Largeness runs in the family—you should have seen his grandfather," as if these were good enough excuses to stay fat for life. The truth is probably that the entire clan was fat simply because they all ate too much, had always done so, and therefore thought it quite normal. Cancerians are not the most energetic of people, and where lack of exercise and the wrong diet coupled with emotional stress co-exist those of this sign are prone to another typical problem: constipation. The Cancerian diets given later have been compiled bearing in mind the physical aspects of these problems, but of course it is difficult to ease the emotional causes; however, if Cancerians feel they must eat when someone has slighted them they should try to make it an apple or a piece of chewing-gum rather than a box of chocolates. Better still, keep busy and refuse to sit around feeling sorry for yourself. And, given your reluctance to splash out large sums of money on expensive clothes, why not do just that—buy something you'd love to wear, no matter how impractical, in the size you'd like to be. Then hang it on the outside of your wardrobe as a daily reminder and an incentive for you to lose those surplus inches.

WHAT KIND OF DIET?

Those born under the sign of Cancer tend to lack sufficient calcium; the importance of this is apparent when it is stated that over fifty per cent of the bony structure of the body is made up of calcium. So you may be badly affected by any deficiency of this element in your diet and may suffer from conditions such as varicose veins, haemorrhoids, prolapses and in extreme cases weakened eyesight. It is best to take calcium in its natural food form, for non-natural calcium preparations often irritate the delicate organisms. The following are rich sources of calcium: cabbage (savoy or red), watercress, milk, prunes, cottage cheese, onions. Other foods valuable to the Cancerian are: parsley, oranges, lemons, chives, dandelions, raisins, leek leaves, egg yolk, and rye bread.

SPECIAL CANCERIAN RECIPES

The following recipes are ideal for when the Cancerian is feeling sickly or run down.

Onion and Cottage Cheese Spread
Mix both ingredients together and spread on a rye biscuit or piece of wholemeal bread.

Cancerian Cocktail
Mix equal quantities of milk and carrot juice and allow the mixture
to stand for an hour before serving. This makes a refreshing drink.

Cancerian Soup
Chop and fry 2 small onions in a little fat. Wash and shred a small
spring cabbage and place in a stewpot with the onions and 3 pints
of water. Bring to the boil, then simmer for 2 hours. Add ½ pint of
milk and simmer for another 10 minutes. Season to taste and serve
with dry toast.

THE SEVEN-DAY CANCERIAN DIET

Monday

Breakfast:	½ cup dried apricots
	1 toasted slice wholemeal bread, with ½ oz butter
	1 cup tea or coffee, no sugar
Lunch:	4 tablespoons cottage cheese
	2 oz cucumber
	2 tablespoons grated carrots
	½ glass buttermilk or yogurt
Dinner:	2 slices lean beef
	½ cup beetroot
	½ cup grated onion and carrot
	1 tomato
	1 large orange
	1 oz buttermilk

Tuesday

Breakfast:	½ cup crushed orange mixed with 1 oz lemon juice
	1 boiled egg
	1 piece of wholemeal bread, no butter
	1 cup tea or coffee, no sugar
Lunch:	3 oz Cheddar cheese with watercress and lettuce
	1 tomato, sprinkled with lemon juice and parsley
	½ cup raspberries or loganberries
	½ cup buttermilk
Dinner:	2 poached eggs on 1 slice wholemeal bread
	½ cup leafy vegetables
	1 oz hazelnuts
	1 large peach
	1 cup skimmed milk

Wednesday

Breakfast: 1 glass lemon or Cancerian Cocktail
               1 scrambled egg on wholemeal or rye bread
               1 cup tea or coffee, no sugar

Lunch: 1 medium portion lean meat or fish
               ½ cup brussels sprouts/broccoli/cauliflower
               1 sliced apple mixed with raisins or dates
               1 cup skimmed milk

Dinner: 2 slices lean ham
               1 tomato
               1 stick celery and 1 stick chicory
               ½ cup dates
               ½ cup figs
               1 cup lemon tea

Thursday

Breakfast: 1 glass fruit juice or Cancerian Cocktail
               ½ cup stewed apple or baked apple
               1 cup tea or coffee, no sugar

Lunch: 1 grilled chop or piece of liver
               salad or raw chopped vegetables with lemon juice
               1 yogurt

Dinner: 1 medium portion sole sprinkled with lemon juice
                   and parsley
               ½ cup savoy cabbage or red cabbage
               ½ cup tinned grapefruit
               ½ cup buttermilk

Friday

Breakfast: 1 glass pure lemon juice
               ½ cup stewed prunes
               1 small bowl cereal

Lunch: 1 small omelette sprinkled with 1 tablespoon grated
                   cheese
               small mixed green salad
               1 large apple/pear/peach
               1 cup lemon tea

Dinner: 1 small hamburger
               tomato and green pepper salad sprinkled with lemon
                   juice and parsley
               1 oz chopped onion

½ cup cherries or fruit cocktail
1 cup skimmed milk

Saturday

Breakfast: 1 glass fruit juice
1 rasher bacon on slice of rye or wholemeal bread
1 cup lemon tea

Lunch: 1 slice cheese on toast with 1 poached egg
1 glass orange or lemon juice

Dinner: 2 soused herrings or 4 oz other cooked fish
mixed green salad sprinkled with lemon juice
1 yogurt mixed with 1 tablespoon brewers' yeast
1 cup tea or coffee, no sugar

Sunday

Breakfast: ½ cup apricots or ½ orange
1 scrambled egg and 1 rasher bacon
1 slice wholemeal bread, no butter
1 cup lemon tea

Lunch: 1 small jacket potato sprinkled with 1 oz grated
cheese
1 tablespoon grated carrots
½ cup skimmed milk

Dinner: 4 oz smoked salmon or 10 king prawns
2 oz cucumber sprinkled with lemon juice
1 large sliced tomato
small portion potato salad
2 oz grapes
1 cup tea or coffee, no sugar

EXOTIC CANCERIAN RECIPE

Cancer rules Scotland, Holland, New Zealand and Paraguay, and food from these countries is particularly appealing to Cancerians. So why not celebrate the end of your diet with the Dutch dish below. (Hint to seducers: this dish will go a long way towards coaxing your hard-shelled friend into submission!)

Dutch Mussel Cocktail

2½ lb (1.5 kilos) mussels or clams, cooked
6 stalks celery, thinly sliced
¼ teacup oil
2 tablespoons vinegar
¼ teaspoon salt
3 teacups mayonnaise
1 teaspoon prepared mustard
1 teacup reduced mussel stock

¼ teaspoon thyme
¼ teaspoon oregano
¼ teaspoon marjoram
a dash pepper
a dash Worcester sauce
a dash mustard powder
6 parsley sprigs
1 lemon, cut in 6 wedges

Blanch celery in boiling water for 1 minute. Drain and marinate in oil, vinegar, salt and pepper for 1 hour. Mix together the mayonnaise, mustard, thyme, oregano, marjoram, mussel stock and Worcester sauce, until smooth and creamy. Mix the drained celery with the mussels (or clams) and put in cocktail glasses. Cover with the dressing and decorate with parsley, mustard powder and a lemon wedge.

Serves 6.

HOW DO YOU SHAPE UP AS A CANCERIAN?

1. Do you have a sweet tooth?
2. Do you have more than your fair share of minor ailments?
3. Is tea/coffee and biscuits your normal breakfast?
4. Do you often feel that friends and relatives are ungrateful?
5. Do you feel unfulfilled professionally?
6. Have you had more than two drinking sessions this week?
7. Is your only exercise pottering in the garden? (Perhaps not even that?)
8. Do you think your partner is too demanding sexually?

If you answer "Yes" to more than 3 of the above then you're a typical Cancerian candidate for overweight and also health problems, and you could be acting like a really miserable old Crab!

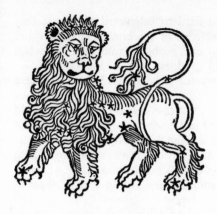

Leo (the lion)

The sign of the king or president

July 23—August 23

The second fire sign:	Proud, generous, trusting, energetic, domineering, authoritative, warm-hearted
Ruler: The Sun	**Gems:** Ruby, diamond
Colour: Orange	**Metal:** Gold

GENERAL CHARACTERISTICS

If you've recently had words with an elegant individual who gives you a dazzling smile whilst muttering "Drop dead," then you've probably been exposed to the Leo. It is not unusual for the lion to display his arrogance and his playfulness at the same time, which is why he gets away with murder. But don't let that soft purr fool you; even the gentle Leo types are inwardly sold on their royal right to rule friends and family, and if you don't humour them their roar is liable to scare you half to death. At least half the people you see out living it up in style will be Leo subjects; shyer pussy-cats will be living it up at home. They go about looking strong, dignified and quietly determined. Subjects of this sign are proud, noble and magnanimous. They wouldn't stoop to anything mean or underhand, and they find it hard to believe ill of others; they are somewhat deficient in knowledge of the human character and this introduces many irritations and problems into their lives. But Leos forgive and do not hold grudges. Just as they trust other people, so they want to be trusted absolutely. Most lions have splendid self-confidence and a good opinion of themselves, but they do require adulation and approval. If they don't find it in the world at large they retreat into a small circle where they are the brightest light. When ambition is thwarted the Leo subject may react by becoming a domestic tyrant and lording it over the immediate family. These types tend to be boastful, convinced that whatever is theirs is best. They are adventurous and can face any danger in the pursuit of ideals.

But no matter how successful, Leo subjects are rarely content. They refuse to accept limitations and so frequently attempt the impossible. Failure makes them very unhappy indeed. The Lion has a magnetic personality and wherever possible should attend to important matters in person, for his enthusiasm is contagious and makes him able to influence others.

The Leo woman is sentimental, and probably owns pictures and mementoes of all her old boyfriends. Chances are she's ridiculously popular—a sunflower not a wallflower—the social leader of her group, behaving like a queen, but with such disarming warmth that no one really minds too much. Anyway it wouldn't do much good to try to usurp her authority. It pays to remember that the female Leo may pretend to be as sweet and harmless as a bowl of cherries; she may have a voice like a whisper, beautiful, courteous manners and a smooth, calm exterior—but she's on guard. Try to remove her as the star of the show and you'll soon find out just how shy and submissive she isn't!

Famous Leos: Princess Anne, Neil Armstrong, James Baldwin, Alfred Hitchcock, Princess Margaret, Mussolini, Napoleon, Jacqueline Onassis, Haile Selassie, Mae West.

LOVE, SEX AND THE LEO

Leo's fiery pride is the cause of plenty of shattered love affairs and marriages; but since forgiveness and sympathy are part of the big cat's nature, reconciliations are about as frequent in the Leo's emotional life as splits. A lion without a mate is a woeful sight; once the fireworks of outraged dignity have spluttered out the Leo gets lonely. This type is almost continually in the throes of passion, not just with the opposite sex but with life itself. Life without love to Leo subjects is like a plug without a socket. Others are drawn to the Leo's kindliness and heartfelt geniality. In intimate relationships with those they love Leos can be loyal beyond the call of duty, generous to a fault with affection as well as material possessions. Without being necessarily passionate they are warm and demonstrative. They like to dominate, yet are capable of great self-sacrifice for a worthy cause or for the happiness and welfare of loved ones.

This type adores luxury. When they invite their favourite member of the opposite sex up to their den, don't expect a cave filled with bare essentials; look instead for a velvet quilt or a fur rug. Leo is very susceptible to the texture of materials and sometimes this can lead to fetishism. The sweet smell of success and its tangibility can literally turn the Leo on. The run up to sexual happenings usually takes the form of an expensive dinner with champagne, etc., for when this type sets out to impress, it's done properly.

One problem is laziness. After some time in a lengthy relationship the Leo individual will be less inclined to bother to put himself or herself out; at this point a bit of stimulation and imagination is called for. But it's worth putting a little effort into a love affair with this type. The Leo man's sexual appetite is well-developed and of paramount importance to him. Much thought will go into affairs and he'll abandon himself heart and soul to each experience. If happily married at an early age the Leo will enjoy a full sex life, growing and developing with his or her partner. Leos are extremely sensitive and are unlikely to become too unconventional or outrageous in sexual matters. If unmarried or divorced, however, Leos tend to disguise their soft centre for fear of being hurt and are quite capable of keeping love and sex separate, and then anything goes, so long as it is experienced in comfort. The easiest way to keep Leos happy is to allow them to believe that their sexual prowess defies description; the Leo who is convinced he or she invented sex will rarely stray. The permissive Leo constantly searches for reassurance and praise in this sphere. Feed the Leo's pride and he or she will always come back for more.

FASHION AND THE LEO

This type's expectations of the good things in life are naturally reflected in appearance. Whatever the financial difficulties, the Leo would rather save up for an expensive outfit than be reduced to buying some little bargain from round the corner; however flattering the latter might look, once it was taken home the Leo would scrutinise it and be most unhappy to realise that it was badly made or cut. Some females born under this sign do let their love of luxury get totally out of control as far as costly jewellery is concerned, maybe wearing four or five large rings on each hand, a series of heavy baubles round the neck and an irritating jangling bracelet or two—in other words, donning the crown jewels in an effort to live up to the regal image.

However, if our Leo subject has been unfortunate enough to gather several unwanted pounds then such ostentation looks pretty ridiculous. While trying to regain a slim silhouette, it is suggested that you leave the family heirlooms in the safe, wear slightly darker hues possibly brightened with the presence of a small gold chain or earrings; if attempts must be made to attract the limelight then Leos should look to their luxurious manes—a visit to the hairdresser and the compliments will continue to roll in. Once the unwanted fat has been shaken off there will be plenty of opportunity to really make an impression confident in the knowledge that glances received are of admiration, not ridicule.

PHYSICAL CHARACTERISTICS AND HEALTH

Leo man tends to have a long, powerful body with short legs and strong hands; a large skull, with a square jaw; thick silky hair; light eyes.

Leo woman tends to have a long body with short legs, and a proud bearing; a wide skull, with large eyes, small ears and nose, and a short neck.

You can't fail to notice the commanding air and stately bearing of all Leos as they gaze down upon other mere mortals. Ordinarily this sign is deliberate of speech and movement; Leos seldom talk or even walk quickly, and they cannot for long be ignored. They'll get the centre of the stage with dramatic statements and action, or else by pouting and sulking until someone rushes over to ask what's wrong.

This sign produces more than its fair share of blue eyes, though many of its subjects, especially the females, have dark brown eyes that are at first soft and gentle then snap and crackle with fire, and are often round in shape and slightly tilted at the corners. The typical Leo mane of hair is dark or reddish blonde and wavy, and may be worn either in a wild, careless style, swept up so that it stands out fully on the top and sides, or else tightly sleeked down at the other extreme. Generally the Leo complexion is noticeably ruddy.

Leo rules the heart, the spine and the back, and if its subjects are not careful their enormous vitality and great expenditure of energy can put too much strain on the heart. However the constitution is normally strong for the Leo has great recuperative powers that easily throw off illness; the likelihood is that this type either radiates vitality or is forever on the sick list. Discordant or

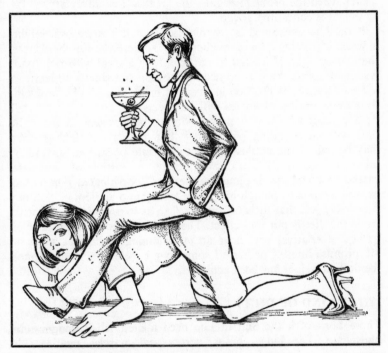

When her ego is deflated the Leo shape is soon inflated

unharmonious environment, hurt pride or unrequited love can all react on the health. The best medicine is peace and harmony.

CAUSES OF LEONINE OBESITY AND HOW TO COPE

The Leo individual, like the Cancerian, requires an audience, and is also particularly drawn to status symbols and anything that can be identified with success. Because of this the Leo loves to entertain and is an excellent host or hostess; an abundance of food and drink can usually be located in the Leo home. On its own, of course, this would be insufficient to cause any anxiety regarding the waist measurement. But Leos need someone to aim a constant stream of compliments in their direction, and when they believe they have been particularly clever in reaching some objective or achievement they can become quite demanding in this. When satisfaction in this isn't achieved then Leo subjects reward themselves constantly—usually in the form of something nice to eat or drink. That's when the problem begins: the greatest Leo adversary, as far as weight is concerned, is ego.

If the Leo concerned is anything up to half a stone overweight, a week of dieting plus a modicum of common sense should put the matter right. If invited to participate in a meal with rich food, wine and spirits there is no need to abstain but simply to learn to use moderation. If the Leo in question has a more bulky problem, then more drastic measures will be necessary. The cure may well be a partner who can tirelessly offer verbal rewards at the right time without sounding patronising; but finding the right partner may be one of the hardest things to put into operation. Instead of taking refuge in an extra large vodka or portion of chocolate gateau to boost the flagging morale, our poor bloated lion would be well advised to plough his or her money into an item of clothing —possibly just that little bit too small so as to provide an objective while the diet is put into effect. The Leo type should steer clear of friends or relatives who have an undermining effect, and, most of all, promise himself or herself some long coveted possessions once the desired weight has been achieved.

WHAT KIND OF DIET?

Those born with the Sun in Leo need a diet rich in magnesium phosphate. The lungs, brain, nerves and muscles require this element in order to function properly; magnesium promotes all building in nerve tissue and lung substances, as well as helping to maintain normal blood pressure. It has an alkaline reaction which assists in promoting an alkaline balance of the body fluids. These conditions give greater elasticity to the tissues and give the joints more flexibility. Foods rich in magnesium are: plums, wheat bran, peas, oats, cocoa, savoy cabbage, oranges, lemons, lettuce. The Leo subject is advised to consciously ensure that the diet is rich in these.

As Leo rules the heart, an organ through which blood from all parts of the body passes, it is essential to keep the blood in the best condition possible. A necessary ingredient for healthy blood is iron, and deficiency can lead to listlessness. This is the mineral that makes red blood and increases vitality, and the Leonine diet on the following pages takes into account these health requirements.

Once two or three weeks have elapsed and the diet has been religiously adhered to, then it is permissible to revitalise it by inserting a day from one of the other signs—a fellow fire sign such as Aries or Sagittarius is suggested.

SPECIAL LEONINE RECIPES

These recipes, which are designed to promote good health rather than loss of inches, will be particularly beneficial to the Leo who is feeling run down, tired or tense.

Plums with Bran
Peel and stone some ripe plums. Mash them well and lightly sprinkle with All Bran.

Leonine Biscuits
Take 2 cupfuls of wholemeal flour and 2 of bran, the grated rind of a small lemon, 1 tablespoonful of honey and 4 oz vegetable fat. Mix well together with sufficient water to form a stiff dough. Roll out on a floured board, cut into any shape desired and bake in a hot oven until lightly browned.

Leonine Purée
Simmer garden peas gently in a little vegetable stock until tender, adding a little garden mint. Rub the peas through a fine sieve and to the purée add a little milk or cream. Serve with cold wholemeal toast, buttered when cold.

THE SEVEN-DAY LEONINE DIET

Monday

Breakfast:	1 glass grapefruit juice mixed with 1 dessertspoonful brewers' yeast
	1 cup mashed plums lightly sprinkled with bran
	1 cup tea or coffee, no sugar
Lunch:	3-4 oz shrimps, with mixed green salad
	1 cup tomato juice/coffee or tea, no sugar
Dinner:	1 large slice grilled sole or halibut
	1 cup spring greens or broccoli

6 dates or 1 large apple
1 glass lemon tea

Tuesday

Breakfast: 1 glass fruit juice mixed with 1 spoonful brewers'
      yeast
      1 poached egg on 1 slice wholemeal toast
      1 cup tea or coffee, no sugar

Lunch: 1 jacket potato
      ½ cup peas
      1 large tomato
      2 oz Cheddar cheese
      1 banana or yogurt
      1 cup lemon tea

Dinner: 4 oz cold chicken, with mixed green salad
      1 peach, well mashed and sprinkled with bran
      1 cup buttermilk/tea or coffee, no sugar

Wednesday

Breakfast: 1 glass fruit juice
      1 grilled kipper
      1 slice wholemeal or rye bread, no butter
      1 cup black coffee

Lunch: 2 cups light soup
      1 glass yogurt, stirred with cinnamon or black
       molasses
      1 cup lemon tea

Dinner: 1 lean pork chop
      ½ cup brussels sprouts
      ½ cup peas
      1 large orange
      1 cup tea or coffee, no sugar

Thursday

Breakfast: 1 glass orange juice
      small bowl cereal sprinkled with wheatgerm
      1 cup black coffee

Lunch: Small omelette filled with 1 oz cheese and 1 tomato
      green salad
      1 large apple
      1 glass buttermilk

Dinner:	2 oz liver sausage
	2 sticks celery
	2 oz carrots
	1 lettuce heart sprinkled with lemon juice
	½ cup figs or dates
	1 cup lemon tea

Friday

Breakfast:	1 small bowl cereal
	½ cup raspberries or prunes
	1 cup tea or coffee, no sugar
Lunch:	Mixed green salad with 3 tablespoons cottage cheese
	1 large pear
	1 cup tea or coffee, no sugar
Dinner:	2 lamb kidneys
	½ cup green beans
	½ cup mushrooms
	½ cup rhubarb
	1 cup black coffee

Saturday

Breakfast:	1 glass fruit juice with 1 dessertspoonful brewers' yeast
	1 scrambled egg on 1 slice wholewheat toast
	1 cup tea or coffee, no sugar
Lunch:	2 slices veal
	½ cup boiled rice
	½ cup grilled mushrooms
	½ cup mashed prunes sprinkled with bran
	1 glass buttermilk
Dinner:	Medium portion lean meat or fish
	½ cup brussels sprouts
	½ cup peas or cauliflower
	½ cup fruit cocktail
	1 cup black coffee, no sugar

Sunday

Breakfast:	1 glass orange juice
	1 rasher grilled bacon on 1 slice wholemeal or rye bread
	1 cup tea or coffee, no sugar

Lunch: Medium serving cold chicken
                  ½ cup cauliflower cheese
                  ½ cup strawberries sprinkled with lemon juice
                  1 cup tea or coffee, no sugar
Dinner: Medium serving salt-water fish
                  ½ cup grilled or stewed tomato
                  1 small jacket potato sprinkled with parsley
                  ½ cup apricots
                  1 cup lemon tea

EXOTIC LEONINE RECIPES

Leo rules France, Italy, Sicily and Rumania and therefore food
from these places will be much appreciated by members of this
sign. One of the French dishes below will be the ideal treat for
you once you have ended your diet. (Hint to seducers: either of
these dishes should help you get that lazy Lion off his tail!)

Quiche Lorraine (Ham and cheese pie)

¼ lb (110 grams) shredded Gruyère cheese | 3 egg yolks
1 tablespoon finely chopped onion | 1 whole egg
½ teacup finely diced smoked ham | 1 pinch of salt
1 9-inch pie crust, partially cooked | ½ teaspoon dry mustard
1 teaspoon Dijon mustard | 1 dash cayenne pepper
1¾ teacups light cream, scalded

Combine cheese, onion and ham. Spread over bottom of partially
cooked pastry shell. Combine egg yolks and whole egg, salt and
mustards. Beat until well blended. Beat in scalded cream. Pour over
cheese mixture. Bake about 30 minutes at 375°F or until knife
inserted in centre of pie comes out clean.

Salade Niçoise

3 teacups potatoes, cooked and sliced | 1 teaspoon salt
3 teacups green beans, cooked and cut in 1-inch pieces |
2 cans (4½ oz each) tuna fish, drained | ¼ teaspoon white pepper
juice from tuna fish | 2 teaspoons Dijon mustard
¼ teacup olive oil | romaine lettuce leaves
¼ teacup wine vinegar | 2 tomatoes, quartered
capers | 1 can black olives, pitted
| tarragon leaves (optional)

Mix potatoes, green beans and tuna fish in a large bowl. To make the dressing, mix juice drained from tuna with olive oil, vinegar, salt, pepper and mustard. Pour dressing over salad and toss lightly until well blended.

Arrange a circle of romaine leaves in a salad bowl. Make a mound of the salad in the bowl. Decorate with tomato quarters. Top with black olives. Put a few capers on top of salad and garnish with a sprig of fresh tarragon, if desired.

HOW DO YOU SHAPE UP AS A LEO?

1. Do you suffer from back problems?
2. If guests arrived unexpectedly, would you have enough food in the house to feed them?
3. Do you think that exercising is undignified?
4. Do you suffer from palpitations?
5. Do you try to keep a good supply of alcoholic beverages at home?
6. Do you feel unappreciated by your mate?
7. Do you entertain more than twice a week?
8. Has it been more than 6 months since you made love anywhere other than in bed?

If you had more than 3 "Yes" answers, then you are not only a Lion heading for overweight but also for health problems, and I bet you're as jumpy as a cat.

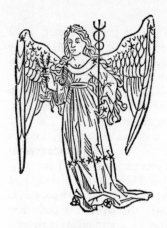

Virgo (the virgin)
The sign of the craftsman or critic

August 24—September 23

The second earth sign: Exact, methodical, industrious
discriminating, intelligent, chaste
Ruler: Mercury   **Gems:** Pink jasper, hyacinth
Colours: Grey or navy blue   **Metal:** Quicksilver

GENERAL CHARACTERISTICS

The first impression typical Virgoans give is that there is a serious problem on their mind that they are struggling to solve. Worry comes naturally to this sign; one might even say Virgoans are affectionately attached to the habit. The delightful smile will always seem to be hiding some great trouble.

This sign is unquestionably dependable and sincere, fastidious in grooming or eating, exacting in work or romance. Virgoans on the move are sure to travel with something of a portable pharmacy, and may need an extra suitcase for their bottles of pills and special soaps and lotions. Vulgarity, stupidity or carelessness annoys them and then they can suddenly become quite nervous and scolding. But the rest of the time they are gentle people and nice to have around.

This is the sign of the critic; the Virgoan can split hairs until he drives you wild. However, if you're in a jam he'll quickly step in to help put things right. It's not ego that makes him itch to take over when things are in a shambles; it's just that his orderly, mercurial mind cannot stand procrastination, neglect or confusion of purpose. Virgoans are practical and down-to-earth. They are diligent workers with competent, discriminating intellects. They are scientific, perceptive and alert. They analyse everything, and to others it may seem they are constantly finding fault. In reality, no harm is intended; Virgoans simply like to categorise and see each thing in comparison with everything else. They are methodical and good at routine work, but need to be careful not to become so obsessed with details that they don't see the wood for the trees. Quick to take advantage of opportunities in commercial concerns, they are thrifty with money and their bank books invariably balance accurately.

Virgoans are modest and unassuming, content to stay in the background. They don't seek constant companionship, and frequently wish to be alone. For the most part they are so cool and evenly balanced that they may never lose their temper. They are content to work quietly and unpretentiously at their chosen tasks, but because they are so retiring—basically shy—they often fail to inspire confidence in others, although with those who know them well they may be less reserved.

The Virgoan female is not the type to climb on a soap-box to make speeches and it would be unusual to find her working in a strip show. But she will determinedly use all her wiles and weapons to pursue happiness wherever its path leads her; a few trips along the way won't cause her to faint or cry weakly for help. She is a perfectionist, with a dogged belief that no one can do things as efficiently as she; and, indeed, usually no one can. She is a stickler for promptness. She won't rage or storm when she is upset, but she can be shrewish and fussy if annoyed. Never forget that this sign typifies the nagger. A clarity of vision will spot an elaborate lie by the smoothest of talkers, and she won't miss the faintest smear of lipstick on the edge of her man's collar. She may be pure-minded but she is certainly not naïve. Hard to please as she may be, it's usually worth the effort.

Famous Virgoans: Maurice Chevalier, Sean Connery, Queen Elizabeth I, Greta Garbo, Goethe, Lyndon Johnson, Peter Sellers, George Wallace.

LOVE AND THE VIRGOAN

Very often, Virgoans' affections are diverted into intellectual challenge. When they fail to find personal love they will instead dedicate themselves to a worthy cause that enlists mind more than emotions. They can be invaluable to humanity; for instance, some of the finest medical staff are born under this sign.

Virgoans tend to be somewhat aloof and solitary; because they keep people at a distance they have more acquaintances than close friends, preferring to divide their affections among many. They are considerate but never wholeheartedly in love. This type can be detached enough to break lots of hearts with a cool kind of flirting. But the critical analytical sense and the fastidious discrimination seldom allow excursions into the passionate. They prefer not to leave the platonic area, so a relationship really has to burn with white heat to produce ardour in these subjects. When they do love, Virgoans may be too practical and are unlikely to sweep others off their feet. This type takes his or her precious time about finding a love object. There may be an occasional fall into an earthy physical experience, but such indiscretions are the exception. There is something chaste about Virgoans, even in the midst of passion.

Virgoan lovers rarely hold illusions and cannot be fooled by lies. They want a decent, honest and genuine relationship, and although they know how small the chances of finding it are, it's difficult for them to settle for anything less. It's not easy for the Virgoan in love to express himself or herself as fully as might be wished, but once committed to a partner the Virgoan revels in devotion. The partner will need to be kind and understanding, for when it comes to sex it is tempting to label the Virgoan as cold. This is not necessarily so. Sex is not top on the list of priorities, but love is reflected in day-to-day behaviour, and during a crisis the Virgoan shows remarkable presence of mind. This type asks and expects little for himself or herself sexually, but tries to make the partner happy. Unfaithfulness is unlikely to make the Virgoan hysterical, and all in all this individual makes a reliable spouse, and a parent who does not spoil a child but offers a sense of security.

FASHION AND THE VIRGOAN

This sign often displays a skill at handicrafts, finding ingenious uses for the most unlikely things, so the Virgo woman is likely to make much of her own wardrobe. Her dress sense leans towards the good but simple, sometimes verging on the puritanical. If somewhat conservative, Virgoans are well turned out, meticulous dressers. Maurice Chevalier would rather have been caught without a song than without his buttonhole and tie-pin. Virgoans are very critical of their appearance and fussy in the extreme about how they look both in photographs and in person. You may catch them creeping in front of a mirror when no one is watching.

Advice on how to disguise superfluous inches is unnecessary in this instance since Virgoans already know that darker shades and plain styles are the best way to go. Having regained a slim figure, however, our Virgoan friend should be a little more daring in following fashion. Members of this sign have a natural modesty and sometimes lack self-confidence, and if they can be persuaded that a litle dash in apparel would do wonders for their ego then perhaps Virgoans would not feel quite so frustrated.

PHYSICAL CHARACTERISTICS AND HEALTH

The typical Virgo man has a wiry frame with bony shoulders and fingers; fine, often thinning hair; a long nose, receding chin, and bright twinkling eyes.

The Virgoan woman tends to have a thin body, slim legs and small feet; square shoulders; a long head, with almond-shaped eyes, a narrow nose and a wide mouth.

Virgoan eyes are often astonishingly clear, sparkling with intelligence and clarity of thought. There is a purity and tranquillity of expression in their faces that belies their secret worries. Most of them are extremely attractive, with delicate, somewhat elongated noses, beautiful ears and lips. There is certainly no lack of charm or grace in this type, and there may be a bit of vanity that pops up at odd moments. The Virgoan is generally quite small, certainly no giant, though more muscular and with far more strength than the fragile appearance suggests. They can stand more intense work over a long period of time than the tougher, brawnier signs, if they can avoid nervous breakdown in the process. Although outwardly capable and cool, any anxieties gnaw away at these types, upsetting their digestion and emotional balance. Virgoans are surprisingly healthy unless worried into illness through overwork, mental tension and pessimism. Straining themselves to breaking point to fulfil obligations may lie behind many Virgoans' ragged nerves.

They may complain about minor ailments such as upset stomachs, headaches and foot problems, but they usually avoid anything more serious. They should baby themselves whenever a chest cold occurs for they are susceptible to lung complaints.

Virgoans take good care of their bodies and are fussy about diet. Many of them are vegetarians; if not, you can bet they know exactly what to eat and how it should be cooked. Nervous skin problems of all descriptions may attack Virgoans, but most health hazards are minor, or else psychosomatic. Whatever the indications to the contrary, this is basically a healthy specimen.

CAUSES OF VIRGOAN OBESITY AND HOW TO COPE

Fat Virgoans are usually pretty thin on the ground, for this sign is conscious of food intake and is also inclined to participate in physical exercise. This type's insecurity is generally tied up with the

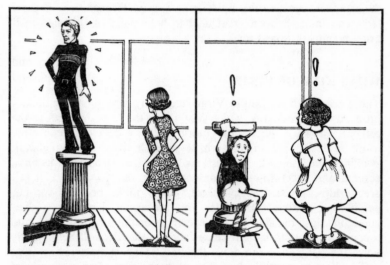

When disillusioned, the Virgoan seeks solace in food

materialistic; most Virgoans harbour a serious debt or financial uncertainty. When totally preoccupied with acquiring money they forget to keep up with physical fitness, and then it's only a matter of time before the muscles turn to flab. And of course while this individual stays up into the small hours trying to juggle the budget, he or she will be instinctively drawn to seek consolation in the kitchen.

An overweight Virgoan, then, is probably someone with considerable financial difficulties. So first of all, instead of ignoring the bills piling up on the desk in order to avoid the unpleasant news, the Virgoan must come face to face with the problem; it may well be that less is owed than he or she imagines. Once the worst is out in the open, a considerable weight will have been lifted from the Virgoan's shoulders, even though in effect the situation hasn't changed. Secondly, since this is an energetic type until depression brings neglect, he or she should resume physical exertions. Thirdly, because Virgo is ruled by the same planet as Gemini, i.e. Mercury, its members have incredibly active minds, so it is important that the Virgoan intellect is kept occupied.

Disillusion is another common reason why Virgoans compensate through food. This type may put some other person on a pedestal, and when inevitably the person concerned comes crashing down the Virgoan feels bitter, cynical and thoroughly wretched—and fills the stomach because the heart is so empty. Recognition of these facts can in itself do a great deal to help those of this sign melt away pounds of excess fat.

WHAT KIND OF DIET?

Those born with the Sun in Virgo frequently have the same dietary problems as Geminians, which may mean they are deficient in the cell salt known as potassium chloride. Such a deficiency can often result in inflammation, catarrh, a sluggish liver, swollen glands, swellings in general, congestions, bronchial troubles, asthma, eczema and ulcerations. Foods containing the necessary cell salt are turnips, green beans, cheese, goat's milk, brussels sprouts, cauliflower, lettuce, watercress and pineapple. Virgo is a diet-conscious sign, the sign of the vegetarian or the health fanatic, and a constant effort to include these foods in the diet will help greatly when the Virgoan is run down through worry or overwork.

To alleviate possible boredom with the diet after a couple of weeks of strict adherence, the Virgoan may extract a day's menu from one of the other signs—Gemini is recommended since like Virgo it is ruled by Mercury. In accordance with the Virgoan tendency one day out of the seven has been totally devoted to vegetarianism.

SPECIAL VIRGOAN RECIPES

Cauliflower and Cheese
Mix a little grated cheese with some finely chopped cauliflower; serve on a crisp lettuce leaf.

Virgoan Salad

Arrange some crisp lettuce leaves in a salad bowl, add some sliced red and green pepper, grated carrot and turnip. Tomatoes and spinach may also be added if desired. Pile these neatly on the lettuce, sprinkle with grated cheese and garnish with a little watercress.

Virgoan Cocktail

Extract the juice from a fresh pineapple; then pulp a couple of ounces of fresh blackcurrants and add to the juice. Dilute with a little water, add half a teaspoonful of lemon juice, and keep mixture cool until ready to serve.

THE SEVEN-DAY VIRGOAN DIET

Monday

Breakfast: 1 glass Virgoan Cocktail
1 poached egg on 1 slice rye bread
1 cup tea or coffee, no sugar

Lunch: 1 glass yogurt stirred with cinnamon, nutmeg or black molasses
2 cups tomato or pea soup

Dinner: 2 slices lean meat
Virgoan Salad
small piece of melon garnished with ½ can mandarin oranges
1 glass buttermilk

Tuesday
(Vegetarian day)

Breakfast: ½ grapefruit with 1 teaspoonful honey
1 baked apple with 1 teaspoonful cream
1 cup lemon tea or black coffee

Lunch: 2 medium-sized tomatoes, sliced
6 stalks celery (remove the tough fibres), cut in small pieces
1 green pepper cut in small pieces
½ cup grated nuts
2 tablespoons french dressing, served with above ingredients on a lettuce leaf

Dinner: 1 large bowl soup
               steamed spinach, greens and onions in a double
                  boiler, dressed with 2 tablespoons of nut cream
                  or 1 scrambled egg—place vegetables and dressing
                  in 1 large baked potato with butter
               1 cup tea or coffee, no sugar

Wednesday

Breakfast: 5 or 6 fresh strawberries
               1 yogurt with 1 tablespoonful brewers' yeast
               1 piece rye toast
               1 cup black coffee
Lunch: 2 slices lean ham
               cauliflower cheese
               1 glass buttermilk
Dinner: 4 oz lean meat
               1 small jacket potato
               $\frac{1}{2}$ cup stewed apricots or prunes
               1 cup tea or coffee, no sugar

Thursday

Breakfast: 1 glass prune and grapefruit juice (equal amounts
                  mixed)
               small bowl cereal sprinkled with wheatgerm
               1 cup lemon tea
Lunch: Cheddar cheese on wholewheat bread
               baked apple with raisins
               1 glass lemon tea
Dinner: Cheese soufflé
               $\frac{1}{2}$ cup spinach sprinkled with lemon juice
               $\frac{1}{2}$ cup carrots, with mint
               $\frac{1}{2}$ grapefruit sweetened with black molasses
               1 cup tea or coffee, no sugar

Friday

Breakfast: $\frac{1}{2}$ cup stewed apricots
               1 grilled rasher crispy bacon on 1 slice wholemeal
                  toast
               1 glass vitamin D milk/café-au-lait (half milk)
Lunch: Cottage cheese salad with pears or pineapple
               1 glass milk flavoured with black molasses

Dinner: 5 oz steak grilled with small onion
                  cauliflower sprinkled with wheatgerm and browned
                  1 cup tea or coffee, no sugar

Saturday

Breakfast: 1 glass Virgoan Cocktail
                  1 poached egg on wholemeal or rye toast
                  1 cup lemon tea
Lunch: Virgoan Salad with 4 oz salmon or 4 oz shrimps
                  1 yogurt or fruit juice with 1 dessertspoonful
                      brewers' yeast
                  1 cup tea or coffee, no sugar
Dinner: 2 slices lean ham sprinkled with lemon juice
                  ½ cup grated carrots
                  2 chopped sticks celery
                  ½ grapefruit
                  1 cup black coffee, no sugar

Sunday

Breakfast: ½ cup raspberries or strawberries
                  1 scrambled egg on 1 slice wholemeal bread, no
                      butter
                  1 glass buttermilk or café-au-lait
Lunch: Stuffed tomato with cottage cheese sprinkled with
                      wheatgerm
                  2 sticks celery
                  2 wholemeal biscuits
                  1 glass fruit juice
Dinner: 2 slices lean ham or fish
                  4 oz sliced boiled potatoes, cold, sprinkled with
                      mint and parsley, no oil
                  ½ cup peas
                  1 large apple or ½ grapefruit
Before retiring: 1 tablespoon brewers' yeast or 1 tablespoon black
                  molasses stirred into 1 glass yogurt or hot milk

EXOTIC VIRGOAN RECIPE

Virgo rules Turkey, Greece and the West Indies and food from
these places is likely to whet Virgoan appetites. So the Greek dish
below will be a treat after you have completed your diet. (Hint

to seducers: this little number will surely coax your foxy Virgoan friend into your lair!)

Greek Rice Ring

8 oz long-grain rice
Salt and black pepper
Lemon juice
2 large ripe tomatoes
2 level dessertspoons finely
  chopped chives
Garnish: black olives

8 green olives
$\frac{1}{2}$ level teaspoon each, dried basil
  and marjoram
1 red pepper
4 tablespoons olive oil
2 level dessertspoons finely
  chopped parsley

In a large pan of salted water, with 1 teaspoon lemon juice, boil the rice until just tender (about 15 minutes). Drain in a colander and cover with a dry cloth to absorb steam and keep rice dry and fluffy.

Meanwhile skin the tomatoes; chop them finely and place in a large bowl with the chives, parsley and finely chopped green olives. Blend in the dried herbs. Scald the red pepper in boiling water for 5 minutes, cut off stalk end and remove seeds. Cut pepper into narrow strips; set 8 strips aside and chop the remainder finely. Add them to tomato mixture.

Mix the still-warm rice into the tomato mixture. Blend the oil and vinegar in a small bowl and season to taste with salt and freshly ground black pepper. Add enough of this dressing to moisten rice thoroughly; adjust seasoning and sharpen to taste with lemon juice. Press the rice firmly into a ring mould and leave to set in a cool place for at least 1 hour.

To serve hot, cover rice mould with buttered foil or grease-proof paper and place it in a roasting-tin containing about $\frac{1}{2}$ inch boiling water. Heat on top of stove for 15-20 minutes, then remove the covering and place the serving dish over the mould. Turn it upside-down, and give a sharp shake to ease out the rice. Garnish with black olives and strips of red pepper.

Invert half a grapefruit in the centre and skewer grilled lamb kebabs in a fan arrangement in the grapefruit.

For a cold lunch, unmould the rice ring, as already described, without re-heating it. For a more substantial meal, fill the centre with cooked chicken, scampi or lobster in Mousseline sauce.

HOW DO YOU SHAPE UP AS A VIRGOAN?

1. Do you have skin problems?
2. Have you been short-tempered of late?
3. Has your smoking or drinking increased at all in the past 6 months?
4. Do you lie awake at night worrying?
5. Has indigestion become a regular part of your life?
6. Do you find sex and money problems incompatible?
7. Do you carry any kinds of pills with you to work?
8. Was it easy to answer the above without hesitation?

If you answered "Yes" to more than 3 of the above, then you are a Virgoan not only heading for overweight but also health problems (and chances are you've turned into a bit of a nag).

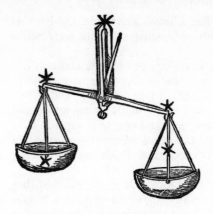

Libra (the scales)

The sign of the statesman or manager

September 24—October 23

The second air sign:	Harmony-seeking, just, lover of beauty, indecisive, charming
Ruler: Venus	**Gems:** Diamond, opal
Colour: Indigo blue	**Metal:** Copper

GENERAL CHARACTERISTICS

Librans are good-natured and pleasant, but they can also be sulky and baulk at taking orders. They are extremely intelligent; at the same time they are incredibly naïve and gullible. They'll talk your ear off, yet they are wonderful listeners. In other words, there's a frustrating inconsistency to this sign that puzzles Librans themselves as much as others. For days, weeks or months on end Librans can be too busy to play; they'll burn gallons of midnight oil, and wash and shine in time to hear the rooster crow. Then suddenly they'll flop into a chair and give the best imitation of laziness you've ever seen. If you try to tell someone who has been exposed to Libran lassitude that this creature is a bundle of powerful drive, you're sure to be laughed at. But Librans know instinctively that to restore harmony to the body they must alternate their active spells with complete rest.

Librans are sympathetic and kind, very considerate and sensitive of other people's feelings. Social relationships are important to them; above all, they need a partner for true fulfilment and happiness. Those born under this sign are usually imaginative and artistic. Their sense of proportion, line and colour is superb. They appreciate music and other entertainments where aesthetic values are involved. They are also fastidious and dislike messy or dirty work.

One outstanding characteristic is Librans' love of justice. If they feel someone has been treated unfairly they will go to any lengths to oppose the wrong, or else will react to the injustice by becoming resentful and cold. When it is a matter of their own judgement they are very careful to weigh all the facts and come up with scrupulously considered opinions. They are, however, so subtly and finely balanced that they tend to vacillate and fail to come to any conclusion at all. They want so desperately to be fair, to see both sides of the question, that it is often hard for them to decide which course should be followed.

Good manners are important to members of this sign, they exhibit them themselves and expect the same from others. Librans are courteous and refined, and are repelled by coarseness or vulgarity. If forced to live in an uncongenial environment they retire into a shell. They are grateful for favours and appreciate kindness shown to them. They may offer criticism but it is constructive and kindly meant.

Libran women in particular will air their wit on any subject with the slightest possibility for debate, and a discussion ends up as six of one and half a dozen of the other. If you refuse to rise to the bait she'll argue with herself, for the Libran can start a row alone, pursue it alone and finish it alone in a grand flourish. Her partner's contribution may be only "But why . . .", but that's all she needs to deliver a brilliant monologue perhaps lasting for an hour. She'll turn on that unbeatable delicious smile every third sentence or so, and her partner will end up changing his mind as effortlessly as she changes hers. One of the Libran woman's biggest problems is her manner of appearing too obliging; she tries not to hurt another person's feelings and the word "No" therefore comes too infrequently or with too great difficulty. She attracts complications and cannot see that the reason lies in her mistaken kindliness.

Famous Librans: Dwight Eisenhower, Gandhi, Dizzy Gillespie, Pope Paul VI, Pierre Trudeau, Ed Sullivan, Gore Vidal.

LOVE, SEX AND THE LIBRAN

The word love is practically synonymous with Libra. If those of this sign did not invent romance, they certainly made it into an art with even more finesse than Leo, Scorpio or Taurus, which is saying a lot. Librans use every trick with casual ease and seldom fail to get the object of their affections. However, once they have triumphed, they aren't always sure what to do with the victim, and having thoroughly charmed him or her into willing submission they hesitate. Should they take advantage of the lover's helpless state, or should they try for marriage? Or both, or neither? The male Libran in particular won't lose interest in the opposite sex until he is ninety (maybe not even then).

Since the art of love-making comes so easily and shockingly early to most Librans, and since they almost always wear the crown of success on romantic excursions, they do tend to get rather tangled up emotionally. They have a horror of anything banal and an inclination towards fickleness cannot be denied, although Librans may remain blissfully unaware of any damage they may do in this way. The natural tendency is to seize up every third or fourth member of the opposite sex they come across, and weigh up the possibilities of him or her being the true soul mate. Librans often get love and friendship hopelessly confused. It's fairly easy to find a soft-hearted, guileless Libra man in the clutches of a determined female who has made him feel that leaving her would be a sin, second only to breaking all the ten commandments. However, most Librans manage to keep free enough to enjoy romance to the fullest. To Librans love is sacred, and they tend to worship the love of the moment. They love with the mind and spirit; few Librans marry for money or possessions.

Because Librans are so refined and subtle in their responses they are often misunderstood and people may react by being afraid of them. However both the male and female of the species are basically charming and affectionate; though they are wary of intimacy on the part of others and can be coldly aloof if anyone tries to presume. If a member of the opposite sex lacks attractive manners, a Libran doesn't care how many other virtues they possess.

FASHION AND THE LIBRAN

The Libran female prefers to dress in silks and laces and invariably her hair will smell of fragrant cologne. She may look as dainty and fluffy as a white rabbit, or even a doll you could lift up with one hand. She's also a girl who can wear a pair of trousers with surprising ease and grace, although she's not the type to live in them. She keeps her ultra-feminine organdie for parties and her slinky silks for her privacy. For the most part she dresses to enhance her typical chocolate-box image, and why shouldn't she? Well, one good reason against it could be overweight. There's nothing more incongruous than a plump female pouting and dressed to kill in frills and bows. Fine when you're a size eight, but the vision of an overblown size eighteen in the same get-up is enough to give the most straightfaced the giggles. I hope our Libran friends have got the message and aren't too offended. Put away that sweet lace number and take out something plainer, without a frill in sight. There's no reason why you shouldn't wear something a little daring, but until you lose weight no slinky outfits, please. Librans are rarely tall, and many in fact are below average in height, so the length of the hemline is most important. Anything too short will make you look as if you are toddling on two pork sausages; anything too long could make your legs seem nonexistent altogether. Just below the knee is the ideal length for skirts until those pounds can be made to evaporate; well tailored dark trousers are also a sensible choice.

PHYSICAL CHARACTERISTICS AND HEALTH

Libra man tends to have a fairly rounded frame, with pronounced hips and thighs; quite thin arms; a short neck and a square face, with cupid-bow mouth and dimples.

Libra woman tends to have a medium build; a curvy figure with largish bust and good legs; light coloured hair; a square jaw, pale eyes and a heart-shaped mouth, and dimples.

Libran features are even and well balanced, pleasing but not always very noticeable, so it's easiest to start with the most noted Libran characteristic: the Venus dimple. There will usually be one in each cheek or one in the chin, and you might check to see if the knees are dimpled—or some other equally interesting parts of the Libran anatomy (but don't blame me if you get into trouble). A pleasant expression is also a marked attribute: even when angry the Libran somehow manages to look mild or at the very least neutral. This type has a sweet voice, clear as a bell, and rarely raises it shrilly or resorts to bellowing. You'll never meet a Libran who doesn't have a beautiful smile, and invariably the men are handsome and the women pretty. Most of them are full of curves rather than angles and even after a strict diet will never quite lose that hour-glass shape.

The biggest threat to their health is over-indulgence of some kind. Eating too many sweets invites obesity, stomach disorders and problem skin; excessive use of alcohol can cause severe kidney and bladder disturbances, which in turn result in headaches or migraine. Libra rules the lower back and kidneys so these are the most susceptible areas. Ulcers beset many a Libran as a result of abuse of the digestive system and the topsy-turvy emotional make-up. Librans are for the most part healthy unless they push themselves too hard. The effect of peace and harmony on them is miraculous. When ill they need prolonged rest with no discordant situations to plague them; pleasant books, soft music and soothing words are the best cure. Fortunately Librans have great powers of endurance and recuperate quickly from illness or disease. An instinct for sanity keeps Librans mentally and physically fit, so that they usually avoid serious breakdowns of body or mind.

CAUSES OF LIBRAN OBESITY AND HOW TO COPE

Although this sign characteristically seeks balance and harmony, yet Librans are known to gorge themselves on food, drink and love-making, throwing harmony out of the window, not to mention completely upsetting the diet. Like the Leo, the Libran likes to socialise, and a madly hectic social life tends to involve plenty of eating and drinking. The Libran shape is often reminiscent of a human lollipop or a caramel sundae topped with whipped cream, and this is just the sort of food these types adore—the thought is enough to make them hungry. A few pounds of overweight can

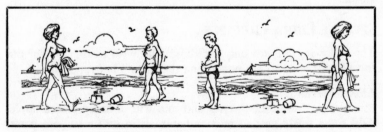

The opposite sex dictates the size of the Libran waistline

usually be rectified by a little common sense, without drastic measures. However, a more acute weight gain probably indicates that the Libran is under some emotional stress. When love passes this character by, compensation begins in earnest and before long those tempting Libran curves become unsightly rolls of fat.

So moderation must be developed, and emotional insecurity must be kept at bay. Librans need a close relationship round which to revolve their existence, and when this is denied them they throw themselves into a whirl of parties and boozing in an effort to forget. To watch them in this state of mind one would think the world food shortage was aimed directly at them, and if this syndrome is allowed to continue until a new love enters their life by then a truly weighty problem will have developed. Once Librans recognise that it is loneliness that causes them to overeat it will be an easy matter to put to rights, for they have many friends. Fortunately this type is extremely attractive and seldom goes unloved for long.

WHAT KIND OF DIET?

Many born with their Sun in Libra have a tendency to be deficient in the cell salt known as sodium phosphate which helps to maintain a balance between the acids and the normal fluids of the body. A certain amount of acid is always present in the blood, nerves, stomach and liver fluids, but any excess is due to insufficient cell salts and this should obviously be corrected in the diet. Some of the foods richest in sodium are celery, apples, spinach, radishes, lettuce, strawberries, pomegranate. Librans should also avoid jealousy, egotism and melancholia as these deplete the nervous system and increase the acid condition of the body.

At the point when the Libran begins to feel a bit bored through having adhered to the diet for a couple of weeks, it is suggested the reader rekindles interest by substituting one of the menus for Taurus, a sign also ruled by Venus and with much in common with Libra.

SPECIAL LIBRAN RECIPES

The following are not only for those who wish to lose weight but for all Librans who are not feeling their usual buoyant self.

Libran Spread
Mash some fresh strawberries and mix with a finely grated apple. Add some finely ground nuts and mix again into a smooth paste. Spread this mixture on sparingly buttered wholemeal bread.

Libran Salad
Chop some young, tender spinach leaves and mix with fresh cream, a small amount of honey and a few drops of lemon juice. Serve on crisp lettuce.

Steamed Celery
Steam until tender some short lengths of celery stalks, and add them to a sauce made from wholemeal flour and milk, seasoned to taste. Add a little butter; mix together and put in oven for 10 minutes. Serve hot.

Libra Juice
Extract the juice from a ripe pomegranate and let juice stand for 1 hour. Sipped slowly, this makes a most refreshing breakfast beverage.

THE SEVEN-DAY LIBRAN DIET

Monday

Breakfast:	1 cup Libra Juice
	1 baked apple
	black coffee, no sugar
Lunch:	1 cup vegetable soup
	yogurt sprinkled with cinnamon or black molasses
	1 cup lemon tea
Dinner:	1 medium portion white fish sprinkled with lemon or parsley
	Libran Salad
	½ cup strawberries
	1 cup tea or coffee, no sugar

Tuesday

Breakfast:	1 glass orange juice mixed with 1 tablespoon lemon juice
	1 slice wholemeal or rye bread thinly topped with Libran Spread
	black coffee
Lunch:	2 slices lean meat
	½ cup green beans
	½ cup cauliflower

                1 large peach, apple or pear
                1 cup lemon tea

Dinner: 4-5 oz grilled steak
                steamed celery
                $\frac{1}{2}$ cup peas
                $\frac{1}{2}$ cup stewed apricots or prunes
                1 cup tea or coffee, no sugar

Wednesday

Breakfast: 1 glass Libra Juice
                1 poached egg on 1 slice rye bread
                1 cup tea or coffee, no sugar

Lunch: 1 small hamburger
                green salad
                $\frac{1}{2}$ cup blackberries or loganberries / 1 banana
                1 cup tea or coffee, no sugar

Dinner: 2 slices corned beef, no more than $\frac{1}{2}$ inch thick
                Libran Salad
                $\frac{1}{2}$ cup stewed apple
                1 cup tea or coffee, no sugar

Thursday

Breakfast: $\frac{1}{2}$ grapefruit
                1 scrambled egg on 1 slice wholemeal bread
                1 cup tea or coffee, no sugar

Lunch: Medium portion lean meat or fish
                4 tablespoons cottage cheese
                $\frac{1}{2}$ cup broccoli
                $\frac{1}{2}$ cup peas
                $\frac{1}{2}$ large orange or $\frac{1}{2}$ cup mandarin oranges
                1 cup tea or coffee, no sugar

Dinner: Medium portion of white fish
                $\frac{1}{2}$ cup parsnips or cauliflower cheese
                $\frac{1}{2}$ cup apricots or blackberries
                1 cup lemon tea

Friday

Breakfast: 1 glass pineapple and prune juice mixed
                1 small bowl cereal sprinkled with $\frac{1}{2}$ cup raspberries

Lunch: 1 jacket potato

green salad
1 apple, pear or orange
dandelion tea or lemon tea

Dinner: 4 oz salmon or shrimps
4 tablespoons coleslaw
2 sticks celery
2 tablespoons grated carrot
½ cup cherries or 1 cup grapes
1 cup tea or coffee, no sugar

Saturday

Breakfast: 1 glass fruit juice
½ tin mandarin oranges
1 piece wholemeal toast

Lunch: 1 omelette, 2 eggs
1 slice tomato
½ cooked green pepper
2 oz cheese with chopped carrot salad mixed with
    celery
black coffee

Dinner: 2 slices lean ham or beef
2 roast potatoes
½ cup cabbage or spinach
1 baked apple
1 cup tea or coffee, no sugar

Sunday

Breakfast: 1 glass orange juice or Libra Juice
1 steamed or grilled kipper on 1 slice rye toast
1 cup tea or coffee, no sugar

Lunch: Wholemeal biscuit spread with cottage cheese,
    tomato, celery and lettuce
1 yogurt mixed with 1 dessertspoon brewers' yeast
1 glass lemon tea

Dinner: 2 lamb kidneys or medium portion liver
½ cup peas
½ cup carrots or cauliflower
1 small piece melon
1 cup tea or coffee, no sugar

EXOTIC LIBRAN RECIPE

Libra rules China, Japan, Burma, Tibet, Austria and Argentina, and Librans will find that food from these countries will meet with their approval. So after finishing your diet, why not try the Chinese meal below. (Hint for seducers: this dish is sure to unbalance that character with the shiny pair of scales!)

Chinese Braised Chicken

1 medium-sized chicken	1 teaspoon sugar
2-3 slices of ginger	4 tablespoons sherry
2 spring onions	3 tablespoons vegetable oil
½ teacup soya sauce	(groundnut or olive)

Clean the chicken thoroughly, and fry it in oil in a saucepan for 4 or 5 minutes. Add one cup of boiling water, soya sauce, ginger, onion. Bring to boil again quickly, and leave to simmer for 1 hour with lid on. Turn the chicken occasionally so as to get it evenly brown. After 1 hour add sugar and sherry and then continue to simmer for another 25 minutes. The chicken is served whole in a large bowl, and cut or taken to pieces with a pair of chopsticks on the table.

HOW DO YOU SHAPE UP AS A LIBRAN?

1. Do you suffer with an ache down the right side of your lower back?
2. Do you loathe sport unless it is of the indoor variety?
3. Would you prefer to miss a bus, train or taxi, rather than run?
4. Do you have a weakness for rich foods?
5. Do you invariably have wine with your dinner?
6. Do you drink less than one pint of water per day? (Excluding coffee or tea.)
7. Is it over a year since you had a romantic dinner with your partner?
8. Are you finding it difficult lately to keep up with your partner?

If you answered "Yes" more than 3 times, you are a Libran heading both for weight and health problems. (And I bet you're becoming an old misery-guts!)

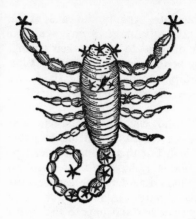

Scorpio (the scorpion)
The sign of the governor or inspector

October 24—November 22

The second water sign: Energetic, independent, passionate, determined, keen likes and dislikes

Ruler: Pluto   **Gems:** Topaz, malachite

Colour: Deep red   **Metal:** Steel

GENERAL CHARACTERISTICS

Scorpio subjects are extremely forceful, with tremendous strength of will. They have compelling personalities which fascinate other people; when it comes to sex appeal this sign is unparalleled. There are two distinct Scorpio types: the higher, represented by the soaring eagle, and the lower, represented by the snake or scorpion. Both types make formidable adversaries, which is evident in their appearance. Sometimes the countenance may almost be ugly, but with a definite attraction for the opposite sex, and even when the disposition is kindly the expression may be stern. The higher type has unassailable integrity, is devoted and high-minded, using ability to dominate people and situations for the universal good. The lower type is sly, secretive and cunning, with diabolical passions. Underhand and treacherous, those of this latter type fly into rages at the slightest provocation. They will take advantage of any weakness and resort to any means at their disposal to wound their enemy. They are totally vindictive, having neither scruples nor compassion for suffering. The more deadly Scorpions will first sting, then sting again, not content merely to even the score but determined to destroy the opponent.

This sign is generally shrewd and energetic, persistent and capable of hard work. Scorpions are tenacious and indefatigable in pursuit of a tangible goal or ideal. For this reason they can be outstandingly successful, though they may have to fight uphill all the way. Because they use their wits, crime detection can be their forte; the lower type can also make a dangerous and wily criminal. Most Scorpio parents are too domineering and impose their wills relentlessly on their children. Yet there can be a haunting sweetness about these people, and gentle sympathy with the sick or despairing. Scorpio subjects are highly selective in friendships, but are incredibly loyal to those they find strong and deserving; they never forget a gift of kindness and it is richly rewarded.

Hiding under the tremulous smile, soft mannerisms and breathless voice of the Scorpio woman may hide a *femme fatale* with fierce powers of retaliation. Hell certainly has no fury like that of a Scorpion female who has lost her normal steady control. She is seldom one to simply like or dislike a person, a play, a book or anything else; she either bitterly resents or intensely worships it. Her dignity in human relationships may make her seem aloof or snobbish. There is an immense store of determination in the nature of this sign, a virtue which can help its subjects out of trouble. It is impossible to be indifferent to Scorpio types. We either love them or hate them.

Famous Scorpios: Richard Burton, Prince Charles, Chiang Kaishek, Aaron Copland, Charles de Gaulle, Indira Gandhi, Billy Graham, Mahalia Jackson, Martin Luther, Voltaire.

LOVE, SEX AND THE SCORPION

Scorpio is the most sexual of the signs; its members love intensely in a physical sense. They are exceptionally wilful and are inclined to go to extremes. If their love is unrequited it changes to hate, and even when their love is returned life is sure to be stormy. Scorpions expect the object of their affections to surrender to them completely and abjectly. They are very straightforward but may be so determined and direct that they frighten the person they are wooing. This is a possessive sign and those born under it must guard against uncontrollable jealousies and excesses of feeling.

Many people find Scorpio subjects magnetically attractive, for they can be sensual and earthy, and no matter how much their lovers give expression to their desires it will never be enough. In the higher types this passionate loving is a noble emotion. But in the lower type it is a gross animal appetite. Despite the fact that many Scorpions can recognise their future mate on first sight, they will often wait and watch before taking the final plunge. They need a mate who is sufficiently warm and sensitive to appreciate that sexually this is an active sign. If the partner can supply all the Scorpio needs as well as remaining faithful, then peace may just be retained; Scorpion types may be compared to a volcano ready to erupt at any given time.

Scorpio women love their homes, which invariably shine with cleanliness, taste and comfort, with everything under control. If the opposite is true then something is making her unhappy and upsetting her natural inclination to beauty and system. The Scorpio woman doesn't go in for blind devotion and doesn't believe in being ardently wooed. She is a human X-ray machine, so unless the pursuer means business he's wasting his time. I wouldn't advise anyone to insult a Scorpion; it's just not healthy.

FASHION AND THE SCORPION

The female Scorpion has a proud, serious beauty and complete self-confidence. Her unconscious regret may be that she was not born a man: less restriction, more opportunity. But once having accepted the difference between blue and pink she'll resign herself to wearing the pink—not that pink is her natural colour. The true shade of her nature is dark maroon or deep wine red, rich colours which allow her to make the most of her lovely eyes and skin. She doesn't walk, she wafts. She doesn't smile, she seduces. And her wardrobe matches her personality. She likes the subtly sexy, the slinky rather than the skin-tight, and can look equally good in jeans or jodhpurs.

Now this is all very well, but what happens when our sphinx has turned into a sow and the wafting is beginning to look for all the world like a wobble? Clearly one cannot shed a stone and a half overnight; it takes time. This is when the focus of the Scorpio magnetism and allure should become the hair, eyes and neckline. Most born under this sign have beautiful hair, and sophisticated styles should now be adopted. Eye make-up can be that little bit heavier and necklines that little bit lower. Loose garments, preferably long, will flatter the usually fairly tall Scorpio female. There is no need to change the favourite colour scheme which is ideal for concealing bulk. The Scorpio subject should make the most of elegant hands, and however possible try to distract attention from the thickened waistline. In fact these individuals have so much going for them that with any luck few people will notice they have put on weight.

PHYSICAL CHARACTERISTICS AND HEALTH

The Scorpio male usually has a big, powerful frame; muscular legs; large square hands; a large head; heavy eyebrows, penetrating eyes, a prominent nose and a strong mouth.

The Scorpio female tends to have a strong, wiry frame with a slim figure; dark, thick, silky hair; well marked eyebrows; strong, sharp features, with penetrating eyes and small ears.

Scorpio eyes may be green, brown, blue or black but they are piercing, with hypnotic intensity. Other people feel nervous and ill-at-ease under this sign's steady gaze; you'll be the one to break the spell and look away, that's for sure. Scorpio subjects have powerful physiques. The complexion is often pale, almost translucent, and the features are clearly drawn; the brows knit together whenever the Scorpion is puzzled. The men of this sign have a heavy growth of hair on their arms and legs, often of a reddish hue. Scorpions walk slowly and seductively. There's a crackling electric vitality about their very presence that gives them away, quiet as they try to be. The poised surface calm of the Pluto character is carefully designed to hide the boiling inner forces. You'll seldom see Scorpions blushing or flushing, frowning or grinning; smiles are rare but genuine. Reaction is kept to a bare minimum with these types so they never flinch with embarrassment or swell with pride; they like to probe other people but remain inscrutable themselves.

Scorpions can destroy the body with excessive melancholy or hard work, but can also build it up at will from a critical illness; such is Pluto's power. These subjects are usually hale and hearty but when they are sick it can be serious. Long rest and a change of attitude with peaceful acceptance replacing burning resentment are the best cures. The chief areas of attack for germs and accidents are the reproductive organs and bladder (where Scorpio rules), the nose, throat, heart, back, spine, legs and ankles. Varicose veins and chronic nose bleeds are common. Scorpio individuals take pride in the length of time they can work without sleep; but when they finally do fall ill they are trying patients for of course they think they know better than the doctor or nurse. These types just cannot put their faith in anyone other than themselves.

CAUSES OF SCORPION OBESITY AND HOW TO COPE

The Scorpion is the true master in the art of excess whose appetites take in anything from food to sex to alcohol, the latter being particularly favoured for self-destruction and escapism. Those

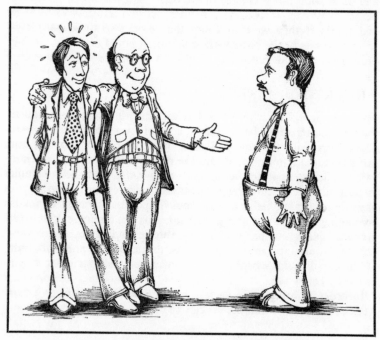

If made to feel inadequate the Scorpio subject overindulges

born under this sign are able to keep life under control while their ambitions are being realised, but if promotion passes them by, or their business fails, they are likely to drown their sorrows in the bottom of a glass. Those close to the Scorpion can be particularly helpful, for this type rarely expresses unhappiness nor asks for sympathy; so if at all possible friends should reach out and give an extra dose of love and attention. Frustration, possibly sexual, may also be responsible for the increase in liquid intake that results in Scorpion overweight, for this type seems to retain fluid. Apart from this, Scorpio shares with Taurus the unfortunate characteristic of gluttony. The trouble is that Scorpions rarely face the fact, and conveniently forget that alcoholic lunch, the Christmas sherry it seemed a pity to waste, that slice of apple pie they stumbled across in the refrigerator while looking for a glass of milk. Apart from business failure, inadequacy in any guise is guaranteed to set these types off on a bout of overindulgence, so they should be extremely fussy in their choice of associates, at least while dieting, and mix with those congenial to their state of mind. However before they can proceed any further Scorpio subjects must stop and think; if they were to count the calories in those harmless-seeming titbits or the one-for-the-road, they would no doubt receive quite a shock, and that's not a bad start on the way to progress.

WHAT KIND OF DIET?

For those Scorpions who seriously wish to get back that slim figure, the first battle must be to retain control over the liquid intake. Those born with the Sun in Scorpio must make sure that the cell salt potassium is introduced into the diet, for they have a tendency to be deficient in it and as a result may suffer from nervous and mental disorders, throbbing headaches, depression, general exhaustion, neuralgic pains and nervous dyspepsia. Some of the foods containing this cell salt are: grapefruit, parsnip, apples, cauliflower, oranges, watercress, parsley, savoy cabbage, asparagus, figs, strawberries, lettuce, spinach, potato skins, dates, carrots and milk. All of these will help Scorpio subjects who are feeling run down or generally below par.

In order to bring some variety into the Scorpio diet after a few weeks, a couple of Aries menus can be used.

SPECIAL SCORPIO RECIPES

Scorpio Broth
Cut up into small pieces 2 medium-sized carrots, 2 tomatoes; add 1 small parsnip, grated, 1 cooked potato and ½ pint stock. Boil for 20 minutes and liquidise.

Scorpio Salad
Shred tender cabbage leaves finely and top with grated carrot.

Scorpio Summer Salad
Slice up and mix any combination of these vegetables: lettuce, tomato, onion, cucumber, beetroot. Sprinkle with lemon juice, and serve with any cold meat or fish.

Scorpio Breakfast Drink
Mix equal quantities of lemon and orange juice and dilute with a little water. For a sweeter drink add a little honey. Allow to stand in a cool place for 1 hour before serving. Add a few cucumber slices if desired.

THE SEVEN-DAY SCORPIO DIET

Monday

Breakfast:	1 glass Scorpio Breakfast Drink
	1 slice buttered rye toast
	1 cup tea or coffee, no sugar
Lunch:	Scorpio Broth
	omelette filled with asparagus or spinach
	2 tablespoons grated cheese
	Scorpio Salad
	1 yogurt with dessertspoonful brewers' yeast
Dinner:	1 jacket potato, with ½ oz butter
	½ cup savoy cabbage
	½ cup carrots or cauliflower
	½ grapefruit
	1 cup tea or coffee, no sugar

Tuesday

Breakfast:	1 glass pineapple juice
	1 small apple sliced and sprinkled with currants and raisins
	1 slice wholemeal toast
Lunch:	Scorpio Salad and cottage cheese
	1 yogurt
	1 cup lemon tea
Dinner:	½ aubergine or green pepper stuffed with 4 oz mince, onions and mushrooms, sprinkled with grated cheese
	1 cup broccoli

1 grilled sliced tomato
1 cup tea or coffee, no sugar

Wednesday

Breakfast: ½ grapefruit
1 slice wholemeal bread
1 cup black coffee

Lunch: 1 glass tomato juice / 1 cup clear soup
2 hard-boiled eggs
chopped carrot and tomato salad
1 glass lemon tea

Dinner: 2 slices lean beef or ham
combination salad with cucumber, cauliflower,
     tomatoes and celery
1 fresh banana
1 cup tea or coffee, no sugar

Thursday

Breakfast: Scorpio Breakfast Drink
1 poached egg on wholemeal or rye bread, no butter
1 cup black coffee

Lunch: 1 cup Scorpio Broth
1 yogurt sprinkled with dessertspoonful brewers'
     yeast
1 cup lemon tea

Dinner: 1 slice grilled sole or halibut (or other white fish)
1 cup stewed tomatoes or celery
½ pomegranate or grapefruit
1 cup tea or coffee, no sugar

Friday

Breakfast: ½ cup soaked dried figs and apricots
1 scrambled egg
1 cup tea or coffee, no sugar

Lunch: Orange and grapefruit sections on lettuce with
     cottage cheese
1 tomato stuffed with grated carrot / green pepper
     with onions
1 small baked potato
1 yogurt with fresh sliced peach

Dinner: 1 slice corned beef ¼ inch thick
                 green salad sprinkled with chopped nuts
                 orange segments with honey
                 1 cup tea or coffee, no sugar

Saturday

Breakfast: ½ cup tinned grapefruit
                 1 boiled egg
                 1 slice wholemeal toast, with ½ oz butter
                 1 cup black coffee
Lunch: Small salad of lettuce and tomatoes
                 mushroom omelette with onions, sprinkled with
                     parsley
                 1 cup lemon tea
Dinner: 1 medium portion grilled trout, sprinkled with
                     crushed garlic, lemon juice and ½ oz butter
                 small raw salad of tomato and carrots
                 ½ cup strawberries or raspberries
                 1 cup tea or coffee, no sugar

Sunday

Breakfast: 1 bowl whole grain cereal sprinkled with nuts and
                     raisins, covered with buttermilk
                 1 slice wholemeal toast
                 1 cup black coffee
Lunch: Large salad of chopped lettuce, celery and water-
                     cress, mixed with ½ cup cold meat or chicken
                 baked apple or apple sauce
                 1 glass fruit juice
Dinner: 1 cup Scorpio Broth
                 ½ small grilled chicken
                 ½ cup cauliflower
                 4 stewed apricots
                 1 cup tea or coffee, no sugar

EXOTIC SCORPIO RECIPE

Scorpio rules Norway, Syria, Algeria and Morocco and Scorpions
will find foods from these places especially pleasing to their palates.
So when your diet has been dispensed with, the Moroccan dish

below should prove very welcome. (Hint to seducers: this spicy dish could well send that smouldering Scorpio volcano into eruptions!)

Moroccan Lamb Roast

6 lamb chops, or rack of lamb
$\frac{1}{3}$ teacup finely chopped celery
$\frac{1}{3}$ teacup finely chopped onion
1 clove garlic, minced
$\frac{3}{4}$ teacup oil
$\frac{1}{4}$ teacup vinegar
2 teaspoons steak spice

2 dashes hot sauce
3 tablespoons honey
1 teaspoon oregano
2 bay leaves
$\frac{1}{2}$ teacup prepared mustard
juice and rind of 1 large lemon
3 tablespoons curry powder

Trim excess fat from lamb. Sauté celery, onion and garlic in oil until onion is transparent. Stir in remaining ingredients; simmer a few minutes; chill. Marinate chops or rack in this mixture 3 or 4 hours in the refrigerator, turning several times. Drain marinade from meat. Wrap bones of chops or rack of lamb with foil, leaving meaty portions exposed. Arrange in a greased, shallow baking pan. Brush meat with marinade and bake at 400°F approximately 20 minutes, or longer, depending on thickness of meat and desired "doneness". Turn meat once during baking period, basting frequently with marinade. For the last few minutes of cooking the meat may be placed under the broiler if further browning seems necessary.

Serve remaining marinade hot as a sauce for the meat.

Serves 6.

HOW DO YOU SHAPE UP AS A SCORPION?

1. Do you seem particularly susceptible to infection of late?
2. Does your work necessitate lunchtime or dinnertime enter-
   taining.
3. Are you finding it difficult lately to keep on top of your work?
4. Have you been too busy during the last 6 months to appease
   your sexual appetite regularly?
5. Do you feel that your ambitions for yourself and for your partner are being frustrated?
6. Do you invariably have an alcoholic night-cap?
7. Does it take longer than usual for you to be sexually aroused?
8. Do you prefer to have a couple of drinks before making love?

If you had more than 3 "Yes" answers to the above then you are
a Scorpion not only heading for overweight but also health problems. I wouldn't like to cross you at present!

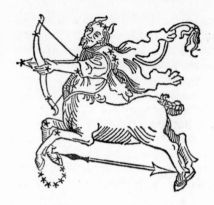

Sagittarius (the archer)

The sign of the sage or counsellor

November 23—December 21

The third fire sign: Candid, restless, impatient, curious, impulsive, nature- and sport-loving

Ruler: Jupiter   **Gems:** Carbuncle, turquoise

Colour: Light blue   **Metal:** Tin

GENERAL CHARACTERISTICS

Those born under the sign of the archer are high-spirited, impetuous and refined; they resent coarseness or vulgarity in others and are aristocratic in their tastes. They are uncompromising in their love of freedom, are very democratic, and have friends in every walk of life. They love company and want freedom of expression not only for themselves but for those around them. They speak their mind, though at times they can be too blunt. Sagittarians' intuition is unbeatable and if they go against their natural inclinations and hunches they usually regret it; their greatest luck comes from trusting themselves. This type has high ideals and true vision, and integrity beyond reproach. Somewhat contradictorily, they can be both proud and shy; they are also quite thin-skinned and easily humiliated.

The typical Sagittarian makes spasmodic thrusts at a variety of things, rather than applying the mind steadily to one project, and once something has been put down finds it hard to resume work on it. However he or she does possess great presence of mind in an emergency and can often solve unexpected situations. Sagittarians love discussion and dialogue and convert others to their viewpoint with brilliant and amusing conversation. They are sceptical about some facets of orthodox religion but are nevertheless very philosophical. The Sagittarian businessman takes a direct approach and is usually successful financially, though he dislikes routine work and is bored by petty details. This is an active sign whose members are capable of great daring, love travel, sport and the outdoor life.

The difference between the legendary Sagittarian straight talking and the brutal speech of the Scorpion is that the latter though conscious of the damaging effect of his words refuses to compromise and feels little compunction about wounds caused. Sagittarians on the other hand are unaware of the possible outcome when honesty compels them to speak out and realisation makes them crushed and dismayed at their own lack of discretion. It would be touching were it not so infuriating. What is in the archer's mind and heart is almost instantly on his lips; he's as earnest as a child—if you want the truth, go to a Sagittarian.

Most of the time Sagittarians are bright, cheerful and gregarious but tempers can flare like rockets if they're pushed about by people who abuse this sign's natural friendliness or get too familiar. Rebellion against authority and stuffy society is also common. This sign is very independent and strangely aloof to family ties, so the Sagittarian female often lives alone. She's also a bit of a clumsy creature; as she strides down the road she may look like a thoroughbred horse—until she trips and lands flat on her face. But even when they break your most prized possession the Sagittarians' disposition can melt the hardest heart and it's difficult to remain cross for long. This then is a sign one must accept or reject; those born under it won't change to suit loved ones.

Famous Sagittarians: Beethoven, Berlioz, Willy Brandt, Leonid Brezhnev, Maria Callas, Winston Churchill, Noel Coward, Sammy Davis, Jr, Disraeli, Walt Disney, Kirk Douglas, Frank Sinatra, Andy Williams.

LOVE, SEX AND THE SAGITTARIAN

Sagittarius is not the most domesticated of signs. It's unlikely that a Sagittarian woman will be exactly ecstatic in the kitchen. But her children will adore her; she'll be their buddy and have a great time with them. Sagittarians avoid marriage for as long as possible, or shun it completely, though suitably mated they can be perfectly happy. A lonely Sagittarian is rare; and the frankness and outspoken attitude are carried through to close relationships.

Though they need to lead lively and interesting sex lives, Sagittarians are not only interested in a partner's body; the partner must also be intellectually well equipped. It's not easy for Sagittarians to settle into an attachment in which allowances must be made for difference in intellect. In addition, jealousy or possessiveness in the partner will quickly make the Sagittarian feel claustrophobic, which can result in affairs and eventually lead him or her to try to break free. There is nothing coy or inhibited about those born under this sign. Their insatiable curiosity results in a tendency to experiment, emotionally as well as sexually; and while this may be desirable to a degree when taken to an extreme there is a real danger of this type losing his or her personality in the confusion. Indiscretion is a common Sagittarian fault which is frequently allowed to accompany these types into the bedroom—it's not everyone who wants to be told how great so and so was between the sheets. However Sagittarians are good lovers; they possess a sensitive ego and would hate to feel they had disappointed anyone. So their partners are unlikely ever to be left frustrated.

FASHION AND THE SAGITTARIAN

There are two sides to the Sagittarian female's image. First, she considers herself the equal of any man and it's not unknown for her to copy her current lover's mannerisms as well as donning his clothes (though her boyfriend's sweater looks a darned sight better on her). However her other side is all softness and femininity. A man with a Sagittarian female in tow will never know whether to expect the tomboy or the sophisticated lady; it all depends on the mood. When the need for elegance does descend don't expect her to trip around in an expensive little black number; she's adventurous and liable to turn up in the latest outrageous fashion (and just as you're thinking she should have been a model she'll topple head first over the coffee table). A slim Sagittarian in her thirties can get away with blue murder, but let's consider the same woman with some excess baggage in tow: the cute little tomboy has become a ridiculous lump and the daring styles look as though they belong to her kid sister. This is often a tall sign and those extra inches of height are certainly useful helping to disguise a few unwanted pounds; but Sagittarians have only to acquire a couple of surplus pounds and their clumsiness has everyone believing they're at least two stone over the top. This individual should now be prepared to make one or two changes in her wardrobe. The jeans and sweater should temporarily be put to rest as should trendy clothes in all the colours of the rainbow. Exciting styles in paler shades should be adopted and (lest she trip over them) perhaps long flowing dresses should be forgotten. Simplicity must be the aim for the time being. Once that fat has disappeared, the weird and fantastic can be resurrected.

PHYSICAL CHARACTERISTICS AND HEALTH

The Sagittarian man is either very tall or very short, with a slim body and long thighs; a broad forehead, often with a receding hairline; bright eyes, a snub nose, and a wide, frank mouth.

The Sagittarian woman usually has a long-waisted body, with good figure and legs; light-coloured hair; an open, honest face, with snub nose, thin eyebrows and a kind mouth.

This type is easy to recognise by the well-shaped skull and high, broad forehead. The features will be cheerful, inviting friendship and the exchange of ideas, and the movements will normally be rapid. Sagittarians often make wide, sweeping gestures that are dramatic and vigorous but not very graceful—they wave their arms to make a point and upset the ketchup. The eyes are alert, sparkling and twinkling with refreshing humour. A stray lock of hair may keep falling over the forehead, like a horse's mane, and will be flipped back with a toss of the head or a quick unconscious hand movement, a habit that may persist long after a new hairstyle has been adopted or even after baldness has set in. Sagittarians are restless; they hate to sit or stand still, and walk as if they are always really going somewhere. The Archer is physically conspicuous if only for his obvious confidence and disregard for conventional behaviour.

Sagittarius rules the thighs, hips and tendons and trouble can be expected from these parts. Those born under this sign are highly-strung so that under prolonged strain they may be subject to nervous breakdowns. But for the most part Sagittarians are healthy and live to ripe old ages.

CAUSES OF SAGITTARIAN OBESITY AND HOW TO COPE

Sagittarians are neither hypersensitive nor particularly dependent on others, so their weight problem is rarely of the compensating nature. Sagittarius is the sign of the sportsman and most members lead an extremely active life; then comes the point when they decide the time has come to retire from the game, and instead they stand eating or drinking on the sidelines and make no attempt to replace

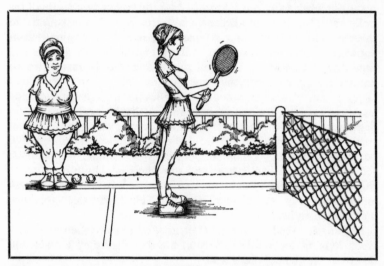

When the Sagittarian's sporting life ends, muscles turn to fat

the energy output in some way. Ideally, when the time comes to hang up the football boots or tennis racquets, swimming or a more leisurely sport like golfing should be taken up: or the Sagittarian should get into the habit of walking to the shops instead of catching a bus. In some cases self-consciousness may prevent subjects of this sign from enjoying the active social life they like so much to be involved in; their clumsy tendency draws attention to the slightest overweight problem which in turn makes them more awkward. Sagittarians must try to overcome this; if you're the type who likes to take long walks, then don't stop. Try to remember the things you used to take part in, in the old days, and attempt to become involved again, though there's no need to go in for strenuous exercise unless you really want to. If it has been fifteen years since you played a game of tennis, however, do take things slowly; just the walk to the court at first might do some good, providing you don't then sit and eat your way through half a pound of chocolates while mentally participating.

WHAT KIND OF DIET?

Sagittarians may be interested to know that they frequently lack a cell salt known as silica which is located in the hair, nails, skin and in the covering membranes of the bone; a deficiency therefore results in weak nails, poor skin and lank, lustreless hair. Carbuncles, boils and abscesses are all beneficially treated with this salt, for in these conditions it acts as a cleanser and surgeon, forcing all disintegrating matter to the surface of the skin and thereby healing and repairing the damage. This cell salt is found only in very small amounts even in foods that are rich in the element. The body requires much smaller amounts of silica than of other elements but it is essential for the maintenance of health and strength. So Sagittarians should consciously try to include some of the following foods in their diet when they're feeling a little low: porridge oats, parsnips, asparagus, cucumber, horseradish, onions, strawberries, red cabbage, rye, wholewheat and ripe cherries. Those born under this sign should try to cultivate calmness and avoid impulsiveness and exaggeration at all times; this will help lessen their appetites and keep them healthy.

Sagittarians tend to live on their nerves, much as Geminians, so when looking for a litle variety in the diet they may extract one day from the Gemini diet sheet.

SPECIAL SAGITTARIAN RECIPES

These will not only help you lose weight but will be particularly beneficial when you are just generally out of sorts.

Sagittarian Asparagus
Wash well and trim the tough parts away, tie asparagus in a bunch and steam until tender. Remove string and serve asparagus on wholewheat toast with melted butter or white sauce.

Sagittarian Cakes
Mash cold, cooked parsnips and add sage and onion. Cut into cakes and dip them into beaten egg and breadcrumbs; fry in vegetable oil. Serve hot and garnish with parsley.

Sagittarian Soufflé

Wash and slice cucumber into $\frac{1}{4}$-inch pieces, peel and cut an onion into slices; then steam both together until tender. Place in a dish and pour over custard made from egg and 1 cup milk. Bake until set, but do not allow to boil.

THE SEVEN-DAY SAGITTARIAN DIET

Monday

Breakfast:	$\frac{1}{2}$ cup black figs or prunes
	1 slice rye bread
	1 cup tea or coffee, no sugar
Lunch:	Sagittarian Cakes (no more than 6 oz in all)
	green salad sprinkled with lemon juice
	1 cup tea or coffee, no sugar
Dinner:	Sagittarian Soufflé
	yogurt or $\frac{1}{2}$ grapefruit
	1 cup tea or coffee, no sugar

Tuesday

Breakfast:	1 glass pure lemon juice
	1 boiled egg
	1 slice rye bread, with $\frac{1}{2}$ oz butter
	1 cup black coffee
Lunch:	1 omelette filled with large sliced tomato and 2 oz Cheddar cheese
	$\frac{1}{2}$ cup grated carrot or chopped onion
	1 large apple or pear
	1 glass lemon tea
Dinner:	1 lean lamb chop
	asparagus
	4 oz ripe cherries
	1 cup tea or coffee, no sugar

Wednesday

Breakfast:	1 sliced orange or grapefruit
	1 cup tea or coffee, no sugar
Lunch:	2 slices lean ham or fish, with parsnips
	$\frac{1}{2}$ cup cabbage
	1 cup fresh fruit salad, no cream
	1 cup black coffee

Dinner: 4 oz tinned salmon or tuna fish
2 oz raw mushrooms with french dressing
1 yogurt sprinkled with brewers' yeast
1 cup lemon tea

Thursday

Breakfast: ½ cup strawberries sprinkled over small bowl cereal
1 cup black coffee
Lunch: 2 slices lean meat or fish
shredded red cabbage
1 large orange, pear or apple
1 cup tea or coffe, no sugar
Dinner: 1 small hamburger with onions and horseradish
small green salad
1 baked apple
1 cup tea or coffee, no sugar

Friday

Breakfast: 1 scrambled egg on 1 slice rye bread
1 glass fruit juice
Lunch: Medium portion of liver
chopped raw vegetable salad, with lemon juice
dressing
1 large peach
1 cup tea or coffee, no sugar
Dinner: 4-5 oz grilled steak
2 boiled potatoes, no butter
½ cup cabbage and carrots
1 yogurt with 2 tablespoons brewers' yeast

Saturday

Breakfast: 1 glass fruit juice
asparagus on wholemeal toast
1 cup tea or coffee, no sugar
Lunch: Onion soup, with 1 slice rye bread
1 cup stewed fruit or raspberries
1 cup lemon tea
Dinner: Mushroom omelette
1 cup savoy cabbage
1 grilled tomato
stewed pears
1 cup tea or coffee, no sugar

Sunday

Breakfast: 1 glass tomato juice
1 scrambled egg with 1 grilled rasher bacon
1 cup black coffee, no sugar

Lunch: ¼ grilled chicken
salad with lettuce, green peppers, cucumber, tomato
½ cup apple sauce
1 cup tea or coffee, no sugar

Dinner: Chopped watercress salad with cheese soufflé or
Sagittarian Soufflé
½ cup spinach cooked with lemon juice
½ cup carrots sprinkled with mint
1 piece fresh fruit
1 cup lemon tea

EXOTIC SAGITTARIAN RECIPE

Sagittarius rules Spain, Australia, Hungary and Madagascar, and Sagittarians usually find the foods of these places especially tasty. So when your diet is over and done with the following Spanish recipe can be a treat for you. (Hint for seducers: this is a dish to make that smart little filly kick her heels in the air!)

Roasted Lamb Alcaina

4 lamb shanks	1 teaspoon rosemary
1 teaspoon salt	4 cloves of garlic
8 slices of thick bacon	1 large onion, sliced
3 tablespoons chopped parsley	1 teacup white wine
4 bay leaves	2 teacups water

Rub lamb shanks with salt and secure bacon slices round them. Place in a roasting pan and around the shanks strew the parsley, bay leaves, rosemary, garlic and onion. Pour in wine and water, and stir. Roast, covered, in 350°F oven for 45 minutes. Skim fat off the juices; remove bacon slices and return lamb to oven for 30 minutes.

Remove lamb to serving platter. Skim off fat. Strain pan juices and reduce to about ½ cup. Pour over lamb shanks.

Serves 4.

Wine suggestion: Vina Pomal.

HOW DO YOU SHAPE UP AS A SAGITTARIAN?

1. Have you over the past few months given up active participation in sports?
2. Do you have liver problems?
3. Do you have a sallow complexion?
4. Do you prefer to dine out with friends whenever possible, rather than at home?
5. Do you see spots in front of your eyes whenever you bend down?
6. Do you feel unable to turn heads any more?
7. Does your partner comment about liking you with meat on your bones?
8. Do you prefer sex in the dark?

If you answered "Yes" more than 3 times then you're a Sagittarian well on the way to overweight and health problems. (And chances are you're becoming an old sour-puss!)

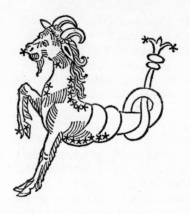

Capricorn (the goat)

The sign of the priest, ambassador, businessman

December 22—January 20

The third earth sign: Ambitious, diplomatic, persevering, reserved, afflicted with deep depression
Ruler: Saturn   **Gems:** White onyx, moonstone
Colour: Green   **Metal:** Lead

GENERAL CHARACTERISTICS

Capricornians—like their symbol the goat—leap over adversaries and obstacles in an effort to climb to the heights. Indeed, they have all the attributes for success since they are hardworking, reliable and have tremendous initiative and drive. They are cautious and conservative, with their own stubborn notions of right and wrong. They are not particularly original or creative, but stick to tried and true methods which may limit their horizons. At best they have a healthy amount of self-respect and are decent and moral; though some born under this sign have the less desirable trait of being obnoxiously self-righteous. Capricorn subjects take life seriously and have a strong sense of duty; they are willing to assume responsibilities, in fact seek them out, but may later complain about how many burdens have fallen on their shoulders. They are steady, faithful and conscientious in the extreme. When it comes to money Capricornians are thrifty; some of them may even be misers. They can be trusted to make sound investments and to account for every penny, but they are not likely to be brilliant speculators; they are too concerned with conserving small amounts to think of making a grand coup.

This type expresses itself rather dryly in speech and writing and may tend to make classical allusions. They are unlikely to sacrifice themselves for others or to give themselves utterly in a relationship with the opposite sex; they are too self-centred and self-interested. They accept the circumstances of their life as a matter of course. While they are ambitious, they usually operate within the hereditary framework rather than choosing a field very far afield; in many ways they feel that what was good enough for their parents is good enough for them, for Capricornians greatly admire those who have preceded them to the top of the mountain and who have laid down the laws of the journey. They court success, respect authority and honour tradition, and are often labelled snobbish and stuffy. Conversely, the goat could call his critics rash and foolish if he were not too wise to indulge in such self-defence. He keeps his gaze fastened ahead, feet planted firmly on the ground. Passion, impulse, jealousy, anger, frivolity, waste, laziness, carelessness are for others to trip over. The Capricornian may glance briefly behind him with pity for the failures, or in grateful tribute for past advice and help, but he will soon continue the steady upward climb until his goal is reached.

Whatever her starting point in life, the Capricorn woman finds the view from the top of the hill most satisfying. There's nothing flashy or pushy about her, but though she may seem docile and apt to contentedly take a back seat to competition, see who gets the promotion. But she'll sacrifice her career for marriage, just so long as she can be a social leader and the mistress of a well run household. She seems to be more even tempered than she really is. Though her manner may convince you she's firm as a rock, the truth is that she's subject to many moods, some really black and long-lasting ones. If feeling mistreated or unappreciated she'll brood for days, weeks or months; her Saturnine gloominess, pessimism and depression is triggered by fear of the future, worry about the present, shame over the past, or a suspicion that she's inadequate in some way. These women do not accept teasing lightly.

When the rest of us need a tower of strength, then this is the sign we should look to. But do remember that when life is bad for the Capricornian it's very bad.

Famous Capricornians: Muhammad Ali, Pablo Casals, Marlene Dietrich, Gladstone, Cary Grant, J. Edgar Hoover, Joan of Arc, Martin Luther King, Matisse, Richard Nixon, J. D. Salinger.

LOVE, SEX AND THE CAPRICORNIAN

Those born under this sign tend to develop an interest in the opposite sex rather later than the rest of us because other things concern them more. They can be lustful and earthy yet at the same time detached and cold-blooded. If Capricornians spend a lot in their quest for a good time, they can be very small-minded and expect the other person to comply with their wishes completely. They are suspicious and touchy about other people's attitudes towards them, for they are afraid of being refused. Once the other person has made the first move, they may feel confident enough to commit themselves but they need every encouragement before they can relax. Should the Capricornian feel rejected, instead of being warm and demonstrative he or she will become antagonistic.

The Capricorn female has plenty of physical desire under that calm, unruffled exterior and it is never satisfied casually. Wasting time on breathless hugs and ecstatic kisses while the future is still unsettled is definitely not for her. When she decides on the right man then the financial situation must be secure. Capricornians don't believe in vague dreams that glide aimlessly through a misty sky; they want to know exactly where the ship of romance is taking them, and that it's sailing on safe waters. Of course there are exceptions who are deliciously romantic, who understand the strange light of the moon and the colours of a butterfly's wing— but they won't let emotion blind them to the facts.

In youth the Capricornian man is an incorrigible flirt, though in later years this may develop into strong protective instincts. Inability to express feelings adequately may be a major Capricornian difficulty. As a rule they are anything but raving sex maniacs and pour most energy into the career; tiredness, tension and pressure of work may stand in the way of the right frame of mind, sexually speaking. Ideally these individuals need a partner who offers reassurance when life goes against them and who can introduce a light-hearted influence into their life. The true blue Capricornian may be a proficient lover but being a conservative at heart is unlikely to try anything at all devious or experimental.

FASHION AND THE CAPRICORNIAN

One of the most typical and delightful things about the Capricorn woman is her natural grace of manner and air of impeccable breeding. She may have been raised in one room in an alley but unless she decides to reveal her origins (which she probably won't) her appearance will convince everyone that she comes from an old-line family and was turned out by one of the best finishing schools. Capricornians have a built-in sense of etiquette combined with excellent taste, and need precious little advice on how to dress. They are invariably attracted by the expensive, exclusively simple and somewhat austere styles, which are just the thing to disguise any unwanted pounds; because of this our Capricornian friend can be anything up to a stone overweight and others around may not even notice.

This type of woman needs to be reminded that fashion can be fun. Even she must find it a trial having to look sophisticated and elegant all the time. Once she has lost weight there's nothing to prevent her experimenting with one or two adventurous outfits on appropriate social occasions. If she allows herself to show a glimmer of leg or a glimpse of cleavage, she mustn't imagine that all those around her will think her wanton. On the contrary, the compliments could do much for her morale. This is the woman who will admire a rather daring number in a glossy magazine while remarking that it would far too naughty/bright/dashing etc. for her to wear herself. But why not? There's no reason why you as a Capricornian shouldn't let your hair down and do something just a little bit outrageous for once. It may be the best tonic when you're suffering one of these notorious depressions.

PHYSICAL CHARACTERISTICS AND HEALTH

The Capricornian man tends to have a lean build and short to medium height; dark, lank hair; a swarthy complexion; round eyes, and a slightly worried expression.

The Capricornian woman tends to have a rather thick-set body, straight fairly greasy hair; a long face, with heavy features and a leaden, almost melancholic expression.

It is not always easy to recognise members of this sign, for they can be stocky and muscular, thin and wiry, or plump and soft. But no matter what the shape the Goat will give the impression of being rooted to the spot. Generally these people have dark hair, dark steady eyes and a swarthy, olive or tanned complexion. There is always a faint aura of melancholia and seriousness surrounding the Saturn personality; none of its subjects can completely escape this planet's influence of stern discipline and self-denial. Many Capricornians have strong feet, capable hands and voices that are even and soothing; you'll probably notice a gentleness that flatters and persuades. This type will either have strong white teeth or constant problems with decay and continual visits to the dentist.

Generally speaking if Capricornians avoid lingering depressions their tenacity for life is remarkable. This type has an iron constitution, nerves of steel and terrific powers of endurance. Capricorn rules the bones and joints, particularly the knees, and there may be trouble to this part of the body. An above average number of colds may be experienced in later life, though this, next to Sagittarius, is the best sign for living to a ripe old age. In childhood Capricornians tend to be weaker, more sickly than other youngsters, but strength and resistance to disease increase with age. Those who wish to avoid sickness should have plenty of outdoor exercise and develop a more positive and outgoing personality; the fresh air, the country and the breeze of tolerance will work magic on the Saturnine health. Nearly all Capricorn subjects have sensitive skin that may develop nervous rashes, allergies, roughness and chapping, enlarged pores or acne. Stomach disorders resulting from incompatible foods and mental stress are also common. It is important that these types remember they are ruled by the mind a great deal more than most people, and if they want to be ill because they're feeling pessimistic, in a couple of hours they'll probably manage to throw up a good few symptoms. But when the Capricornian is in a good mood there is no healthier specimen around.

CAUSES OF CAPRICORNIAN OBESITY AND HOW TO COPE

The Capricornian is an incorrigibly depressive character, and will always find something to worry about but most often the blame can be laid at the door of finance—or lack of it. There's nothing like a shortage of funds to put this type into a black, black mood; this is when Capricornians console themselves with extra food and drink, and by the time their spirits finally begin to lift they have gained half a stone in weight. Since this is not the most energetic sign it is often accused of the cardinal sin of sloth though this may just be a general lack of vitality. Capricornians need to be encouraged to join the outside world, but if they stubbornly refuse to socialise and want to feel sorry for themselves there's little that can be done to help.

It is wise to wait until despondency and gloom have passed before launching into a diet, otherwise it will certainly be a waste of time; if you attempt to diet while in an apathetic and depressive state you will be beaten before you begin. When really down Capricornians can come to the conclusion that the only worthwhile things in life are eating and drinking. In more favourable moods they will enjoy a certain amount of physical exercise, which is totally forsaken as they sink into the depths of despair. If the Capricornian can overcome this particular devil lurking within,

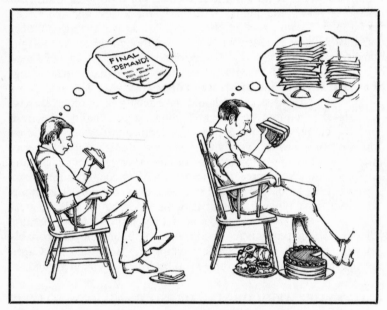

Capricornian eating habits are ruled by money—or the lack of it!

then he or she will have gone a long way towards improving the silhouette. It's also a good idea to get out all those bills, face them and try to see exactly what the damage is, rather than hiding them away in the vague hope that they may disappear. You may find that imagination has done a lot to worsen the situation.

WHAT KIND OF DIET?

Those born under Capricorn are likely to suffer from the same deficiency as those born under Cancer, namely a lack of calcium.

Since at least fifty per cent of the bony structure of the body is made of calcium, a lack of this element can produce bad effects; for example, relaxed conditions of the tissues such as varicose veins. haemorrhoids, prolapsed organs and weakened eyesight. Calcium preparations other than from natural foods are not recommended as they can often irritate delicate constitutions. The following are foods which are naturally rich in calcium and some of them should be included in the diet every day: milk, cottage cheese, cabbage, watercress, prunes, onions, oranges, lemons, parsley, chives, raisins, leeks, egg yolk and rye bread.

In the interests of variety, once the diet has been adhered to for a couple of weeks it is permissible for the Capricornian to extract a day's menu from one of the other twelve signs; the Cancerian diet sheet will probably be the most appropriate.

SPECIAL CAPRICORNIAN RECIPES

Capricornians must try to avoid feelings of discontentment and solitariness, and the following recipes may help when these types are feeling low or physically run down.

Milk Cocktail
Mix the juice from carrots with equal amount of milk, and allow the mixture to stand for at least an hour before serving.

Capricornian Soup
Fry two small chopped onions in a little fat. Wash and shred a small spring cabbage, and place together with the onions and 3 pints of water in a small saucepan. Bring to the boil, then simmer for 2 hours. Add $\frac{1}{2}$ pint of milk and simmer for a further 10 minutes. Season to taste and serve with dry toast or rye bread squares.

Capricornian Spread
Mix together finely chopped onion with cottage cheese. Serve spread on rye or wholemeal bread.

THE SEVEN-DAY CAPRICORNIAN DIET

Monday

Breakfast: 1 glass Milk Cocktail
                 1 slice rye bread with Capricornian Spread
                 1 cup black coffee

Lunch: Capricornian Soup with toast
                ½ can tinned mandarin oranges
                1 glass lemon tea
Dinner: 3-4 oz Cheddar cheese
                green salad sprinkled with lemon juice and parsley
                ½ large orange or grapefruit
                1 cup tea or coffee, no sugar

Tuesday

Breakfast: 1 glass buttermilk
                small bowl cereal with 1 oz chopped hazel nuts
                1 piece rye toast
Lunch: Grilled kidney
                ½ cup spinach or turnip greens sprinkled with lemon
                   juice/½ cup carrots with mint
                2 oz dates
                1 glass lemon tea
Dinner: 1 medium serving lean meat or fish
                ½ cup dandelion greens, endive or 2 pieces chicory
                ½ cup sauerkraut, cauliflower or leeks
                ½ cup fruit cocktail
                1 cup tea or coffee, no sugar

Wednesday

Breakfast: Milk cocktail
                1 poached egg on rye toast
                1 cup black coffee
Lunch: 4 tablespoons cottage cheese
                chopped carrot and tomato salad
                ½ cup strawberries, raspberries or loganberries
                1 cup lemon tea
Dinner: Medium portion any white fish, with lemon and
                   parsley
                1 small jacket potato
                ½ cup stewed prunes or apple
                1 cup tea or coffee, no sugar

Thursday

Breakfast: 1 glass equal amounts prune and grapefruit juice
                2 grilled sardines on 1 slice rye bread

1 cup tea or coffee, no sugar
Lunch: Salad bowl of chopped vegetables, with 1 cup grated
                  cheese and lemon dressing
              1 slice wholemeal bread
              1 baked apple
              1 cup lemon tea
Dinner: Lamb or beef stew with 4 oz meat, 3 boiled
                  potatoes, 1 cup mixed vegetables
              green salad
              1 cup tea or coffee, no sugar

Friday

Breakfast: 2 apricots
              1 slice wholemeal bread with ½ oz butter
              1 cup tea or coffee, no sugar
Lunch: 3 slices white meat, chicken or turkey
              2 tablespoons tinned sweetcorn
              2 tablespoons grated carrot
              small portion jelly with fresh fruit
              1 cup lemon tea
Dinner: 5 oz pork fillet
              ½ cup apple sauce
              green salad
              ½ cup loganberries
              1 cup black coffee, no sugar

Saturday

Breakfast: 1 glass fruit juice
              1 slice rye bread with Capricornian Spread
              1 cup tea or coffee, no sugar
Lunch: 1 jacket potato
              4 tablespoons cottage cheese
              shredded savoy cabbage or red cabbage
              1 piece fresh fruit
              1 cup tea or coffee, no sugar
Dinner: Onion soup with 1 slice rye toast
              medium serving white fish, sprinkled with lemon
                  juice and parsley
              small green salad
              1 cup figs
              1 cup tea or coffee, no sugar

Sunday

Breakfast:	1 boiled egg
	1 slice wholemeal toast, with ½ oz butter
	1 glass pineapple or grapefruit juice
	1 cup black coffee, no sugar
Lunch:	2 grilled kidneys
	1 rasher bacon on slice of wholemeal bread
	1 yogurt sprinkled with brewers' yeast
	1 cup lemon tea
Dinner:	Medium portion lean meat or fish with 3 oz cheese
	tomato and carrot salad
	1 piece fresh fruit
	1 cup tea or coffee, no sugar

EXOTIC CAPRICORNIAN RECIPE

Capricorn rules Mexico, India and Afghanistan, and therefore Capricornians should find food from these countries palatable and interesting. So when you have finished dieting try the Mexican soup below. (Hint for seducers: this dish is capable of turning on nanny-goats and billy-goats, not to mention the odd Capricorn goat!)

Mexican Hotpot Soup

1 large onion	14 oz tinned or dried red kidney beans
1 green or red pepper	8 oz tinned or dried chick peas
2 oz bacon fat or butter	¾ pint stock or bouillon
½ lb minced beef	½ level teaspoon chili powder
Garnish: lettuce	salt

Peel and finely chop the onion; after removing stalk base and seeds chop the pepper finely. Melt the fat in a large heavy-based pan, and fry onion until it begins to colour. Add meat and continue frying over medium heat until it is well browned. Add the tomatoes with their juice, the drained or soaked beans, chick peas and chopped pepper. Stir in the stock or bouillon, mixing thoroughly. Season to taste with chili powder and a little salt. Cover pan, and simmer soup for 30 minutes. Allow to cool, then put through a liquidiser or rub it through a coarse sieve.

Reheat the thick soup before serving. Garnish with finely shredded lettuce and serve with hot garlic bread: cut a white crusty loaf into thick slices and spread each with garlic butter. Put the slices back to the original loaf form, wrap it in foil and heat in oven for about 10 minutes at 350°F (gas mark 4).

HOW DO YOU SHAPE UP AS A CAPRICORNIAN?

1. Lately are you depressive and do your pessimistic moods last longer?
2. Do you suffer with a "nervous tummy"?
3. Is lunchtime drinking almost a necessity in your job?
4. Do you possess more status symbols than your neighbours?
5. Are the times when you would like to do something outrageous becoming more frequent?
6. Do you lie awake almost every night trying to solve financial problems?
7. Do you get down in the dumps for no special reason?
8. Are you often too tense or tired for sex?

If you answered "Yes" to more than 3 of the above then you're probably a Capricornian heading not only for overweight but also health problems (and almost certainly you're becoming a miserable old goat).

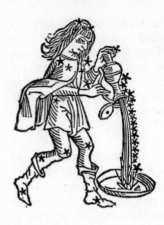

Aquarius (the water-bearer)

The sign of the truth-seeker or scientist

January 21—February 19

The third air sign: Honest, probing, amiable, humane, popular,
broad-minded, kind, detached

Ruler: Uranus   **Gems:** Sapphire, opal

Colour: Electric blue   **Metal:** Uranium

GENERAL CHARACTERISTICS

Aquarians are noble, moderate and stable. They believe in helping
others and are generous and self-sacrificing, without going to
extremes. They have a fine, instinctive understanding of human
nature coupled with great tolerance of human weakness, and a
commitment to the brotherhood of man. They are scientific and
love new inventions and discoveries; often they are very musical.
They are usually well balanced and strong, and their powers of
observation and ability to theorise often amount to real genius.
Theirs is a sound practical approach, in fact their fault may be too
much moderation, for at times drastic action is called for.

Aquarians tend not to be affected by their environment, and
their well-being relies on the mental and spiritual strength they

find within themselves. They approach any problem with an open mind and with such flair that they are ideal people to consult for a safe, sane, well-considered judgement. Their ideas may not always seem reasonable to others at the time they conceive them, for Aquarians look so far ahead that in the short term they can appear wrong; but in the long run, what they predict happens. Once they have settled on a course of action based firmly on facts, they are undaunted by disappointments along the way. They are not influenced by public opinion.

Aquarians do not make friends in a hurry though once they do they are very loyal, and they tend to have a wide circle of acquaintances. Those born under this sign are excellent conversationalists, being intelligent, sensible and well educated. They are likely to be staunch believers in astrology and also to have an interest in psychic research. With money Aquarians are neither stingy nor profligate, valuing money not for its own sake but rather as a means to an end. They make excellent parents; they rarely spoil their children, but give each child the freedom to develop as an individual and at the same time provide gentle guidance.

The average Aquarian girl is a social delight—graceful, witty, bright as a new penny and extremely adaptable; she has charming manners and may be quite reserved. However, be warned: there are some pretty wild, way-out ladies born under this sign; and when those unpredictable Uranian urges strike, a conversation with this type can be remarkable to say the least. You can expect the Aquarian woman to probe into your inner being until you haven't a secret left or a dream unanalysed. But don't you try to dissect her private thoughts; the Aquarian doesn't play the game that way. She'll keep her motives hidden and sometimes take a perverse pleasure in deliberately confusing you. She will usually be truthful to a fault, but then remember that to an Aquarian telling a lie is one thing, refraining from telling the whole story is another. So if you decide to become involved with a Aquarian, prepare yourself for the unexpected. If you like a life full of surprises then this is the sign for you.

Famous Aquarians: Charles Dickens, Dame Edith Evans, Frederico Fellini, Tennessee Ernie Ford, Frederick the Great of Prussia, Abraham Lincoln, Harold Macmillan, Yehudi Menuhin, Mozart, Ronald Reagan.

LOVE, SEX AND THE AQUARIAN

Aquarians are unlikely to settle down with one person. They love all humanity and are prone to being interested in a whole series of people. They seek quantity rather than quality in their associations and seldom settle down to a steady relationship for more than a limited period. They are such profound students of human behaviour that they cannot be deceived by those who do not live up to their high standards. There is little that is passionate or earthy about these types and they are not especially subject to physical attractions. Ordinarily it's difficult to get an Aquarian to make a precise date. This type would rather keep it loose and doesn't like being pinned down to specific obligations at specific times, preferring a casual "I'll see you around". However, once having been nailed down to a particular hour, the Aquarian will be there on the dot.

The Aquarian female has the detachment and lack of emotion of the air element. A happy relationship with her depends on her being left free to pursue her many interests, so don't try to prevent her circulating among her friends. She cannot be tied to the stove or bedpost. Her loving can be tender and inspired but there'll always be a vaguely elusive quality about it. She thinks physical love is pleasant enough if it's not over-emphasised; she is able to respond to lovemaking with intensity, but if you prefer to keep things platonic from time to time then that will suit her too. Despite their fixation on friendships Aquarians have few intimates. This type chooses for a partner someone to be a friend as well as a lover, the latter being inadequate without the former, and is unlikely to be attracted to a person with a keen sexual appetite. Aquarians marry late in life; in order to find happiness they need to find a partner with a similar outlook and not to try to rearrange their mate. Since the Aquarian woman frequently tells herself there are more important things than sex, when she does become involved she prefers to get down to basics as soon as possible, so that she may return to the fulfilment of her many other duties. Because of this, many sexually aggressive women are born under this sign; they see no need for the man to go through the preliminaries and they tend to take over the dominant role themselves.

FASHION AND THE AQUARIAN

The Aquarian woman's manner of dressing can stop the faint-hearted among us dead in our tracks Beautiful though they may be, few born under this sign could grace a fashion magazine's cover, for the average Aquarian is, to put it mildly, anything but conventional. She wears some outfits a gypsy would only envy and her naked individuality can produce some unique combinations. She'll be the first to wear a new fad, no matter how crazy, and at the same time favours her great-grandmother's styles. With typical Aquarian indifference she mixes yesterday's lace with today's jumpsuit, and the effect can be startling. She'll wear an ostrich boa to the supermarket, shorts to the opera, tennis shoes to a formal evening, and may positively drip with imitation diamonds when she visits the funfair. And she's quite indifferent to her friends' opinions. Her originality is her way of expressing herself, and to try to restrain her would only prompt rebellion and cause her to become even more bizarre.

Bearing in mind that suggestions aimed at restricting this flamboyant character may have the opposite effect, I can only appeal to the Aquarian's excellent common sense and logic. After all, a slim and beautiful girl can afford to look a little unusual as a result of her far-out ways of throwing her wardrobe together, but what about that same zany lady with an extra stone in weight? Instead of being able to delightfully shock others into taking notice, something the Aquarian female takes mischievous delight in doing, she will also notice acute embarrassment. There's no point in trying to persuade our crazy friend into a neat little black dress, but I would like tactfully to suggest that the overweight Aquarian might tone down the outrageous styles a little and at least make sure that an outfit in fact does fit. Nobody likes to see rolls of fat trying to escape from a skin-tight dress; and purple thigh boots, bright red micro-mini skirt, shawl and enormous straw hat can make a plump Aquarian look like an unappetising dumpling in a plate of brightly coloured vegetables. So if she can bear in mind that after a couple of months of weight-watching she'll be able to be as delightfully crazy as ever, then in the meantime she'll be able to avoid the uncomfortable position of knowing that others are laughing at her.

PHYSICAL CHARACTERISTICS AND HEALTH

Aquarian men often have quite a feminine shape, with long arms; clean-cut features, with wide-apart eyes, a thin upper lip and small ears; and prematurely greying hair.

The Aquarian woman generally has a slim boyish figure, with small bust and excellent legs; an open face, with wide eyes and a pleasant mouth.

Aquarian eyes are an easily recognisable feature, with that strange, far-away look as if they possess some mysterious knowledge nobody else can penetrate; for all Aquarians' eyes are typically vague and have a wandering expression. The hair is often straight and silky, likely to be blonde, sandy or light brown; the complexion is pale, and the height usually above average. The Aquarian features are finely chiselled and the profile has a marked nobility. One of their characteristics may be the adoption of a pose with drooping head when they are thinking about a problem. Thanks to the dual sexuality of Uranus, their ruling planet, Aquarians often have feminine characteristics in a male body, for instance broad hips, and masculine characteristics such as broad shoulders in a female body.

This type's health is basically sound, but obscure nervous disorders may occur. Aquarius rules the lower legs, ankles and blood circulation, and any illnesses are liable to be in connection with these areas. Subjects of this sign shiver and shake in winter and suffer with humidity in the summer. They are susceptible to varicose veins, hardening of the arteries, pains in the legs due to poor circulation, sore throats and sometimes heart palpitations, but usually not of the serious variety. Aquarians seldom take advantage of the three remedies they need most: fresh air—they close the windows, pile on the blankets and still complain that they are freezing; sleep—because of the high-frequency nervous tension that accompanies their mental activity the rest they do get is troubled by strange dreams; and physical exercise—unless Aquarians develop early a love of sport it's difficult to prod them into moving fast, let alone running along a track. The mind gets a continual work-out but the body needs a strong push. In childhood Aquarians' health is excellent, apart from the odd Uranian complaint impossible to diagnose; their real troubles begin when maturity increases stubbornness. Aquarians' health, then, is in their own hands. Providing they have a sensible attitude and accept the limitations of the body, they will remain hale and hearty.

CAUSES OF AQUARIAN OBESITY AND HOW TO COPE

Having established that the Aquarian is neither highly sexed nor materialistic, we know that weight gain in this type is unlikely to have any connection with these facets of life. This individual's particular demon is frustration. The Aquarian's plans and ideas are usually so far advanced that they may be totally beyond comprehension and receive little sympathy from other people. In many instances, however, these ideas are eccentric and impractical; yet still the Aquarian charges in with plans to reform his or her boss, firm, friends or loved ones. Unfortunately, diplomacy isn't a virtue of this sign, and in presenting suggestions Aquarians are somewhat lacking in tact and naturally such an attitude is inclined to arouse opposition. So Aquarians are frequently thwarted in their desire to improve mankind. Small wonder, then, that their problem is frustration. They are normally logical, open-minded individuals, so

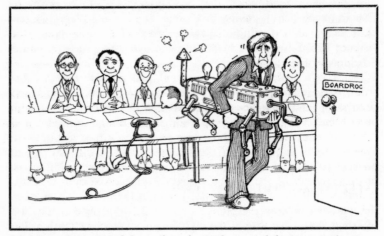

The Aquarian overindulges when the fools around don't recognise his genius

it's hard to understand why it is impossible to point out to them the error of their ways; should anyone try, the opinionated side of the Aquarian character emerges and they become very stubborn. These types are eager to point the spotlight of truth on those around, but are most uncomfortable if the same methods are applied on themselves. So what is to be done when that frustration results in extra pounds? That's a difficult question to answer since the Aquarian doesn't take kindly to advice. But providing he or she can be persuaded to take things a little more slowly and try to be more adaptable, the frustration could be considerably minimised together with the urge to overeat.

WHAT KIND OF DIET?

Those born with the Sun in Aquarius are quite often deficient in salt. When this occurs it means that the water of the body is not properly controlled and this condition is liable to permit the development of ailments such as catarrh, dropsy, diarrhoea, delirium, water blisters. The diet of an Aquarian should contain a certain amount of sodium-based foods and iodine foods. The latter could be described as a beauty mineral, for it is necessary for the healthy functioning of the glands, good-looking hair and unblemished skin. Every time you consume sea food you're getting an amount of this element. Nowadays, sea greens and sea vegetables are being used by many who live alongside the oceans, and in dried or powdered forms by those living away from the seashores. Thousands are using sea salt in place of the ordinary white table salt so common to us all. The following list of iodine-based foods should feature in the diet of all conscientious Aquarians: oysters, shrimps, lobsters, sea-water fish, sea greens, sea-water vegetable salt.

Aquarians' need and love of other people may mean that in the course of the diet they will be persuaded to participate in a sumptuous meal. Instead of feeling guilty, they should embark on the one-day hangover diet, or the one-day beauty diet, which should repair the damage. After this they can return to the diet sheet, if necessary enlivening it with one day from the Taurean diet.

SPECIAL AQUARIAN RECIPES

Aquarian Savoury
Cook 1 cup diced celery in casserole with a little water and butter until tender. Cook ½ cup spaghetti in boiling salty water for 10-15 minutes then drain. Make 1 cup of white sauce. Mix celery and spaghetti; stir in the sauce and ½ cup of grated cheese. Turn into a flat baking dish, put a few dots of butter on top and bake until nicely brown. For a change, add mushrooms, tomato or hard-boiled egg.

Aquarian Salad
Cut a freshly cooked beetroot into thin slices and simply serve with lemon juice or with a small amount of mayonnaise. Place on a bed of lettuce or watercress.

Aquarian Breakfast Drink
1. Plum juice has laxative properties and also contains an enzyme which aids digestion. It is a good spring and summer body cleanser, it helps with digestive disorders, constipation, biliousness, overweight and skin problems. Plum stones should of course be removed before putting fruit in liquidiser.
2. Peach juice is also a good body cleanser and blood purifier. It has a mild laxative action and can be most helpful in cases of

constipation, poor digestion, overweight and high blood pressure. Skin and stone should be removed before fruit is liquidised.

THE SEVEN-DAY AQUARIAN DIET

Monday

Breakfast: 1 glass plum juice
yogurt mixed with ½ oz currants
1 slice wholemeal or rye toast
black coffee

Lunch: 2 slices lean meat or fish
raw salad of tomatoes, lettuce, cucumber, onions, peppers
1 banana
1 cup tea or coffee, no sugar

Dinner: Aquarian Savoury
1 pomegranate or 1 grapefruit
1 cup tea or coffee, no sugar

Tuesday

Breakfast: 1 glass peach juice
1 lightly boiled egg
1 slice rye toast
1 cup tea or coffee, no sugar

Lunch: Small piece melon with 2 tablespoons cottage cheese, sprinkled with parsley and lemon juice
1 orange

Dinner: 4 oz shrimps or 4 mussels or 4 oysters
small green salad
1 yogurt with 1 dessertspoonful chopped walnuts
1 cup lemon tea

Wednesday

Breakfast: 1 glass tomato juice
1 cup dried apricots or figs
1 cup black coffee

Lunch: Orange and grapefruit sections on a bed of lettuce with 2 tablespoons cottage cheese
1 baked apple, or 1 sliced apple sprinkled with raisins or currants
1 cup lemon tea

Dinner: 2 slices lean poultry
¼ cup spinach or broccoli
½ cup carrots or braised celery
1 sliced pear, with orange sections
1 cup café-au-lait, no sugar

Thursday

Breakfast: 1 glass plum juice
1 poached egg on 1 slice rye bread
1 cup tea or coffee, no sugar

Lunch: 1 jacket potato
1 oz radishes, 2 sticks celery, 2 tablesoons grated
carrot
1 cup tea or coffee, no sugar

Dinner: Aquarian Salad
medium portion of salt-water fish
yogurt sprinkled with 1 tablespoon brewers' yeast
1 cup lemon tea

Friday

Breakfast: 1 glass peach juice
1 poached egg, 1 rasher grilled bacon
1 slice wholemeal bread, no butter
1 cup black coffee

Lunch: Medium portion liver
½ cup green beans
1 sliced tomato
1 cup lemon tea

Dinner: 2-egg omelette, with 1 oz sliced mushrooms, 1 small
onion chopped finely
2 boiled potatoes
1 large pear or apple
1 cup tea or coffee, no sugar

Saturday

Breakfast: 1 glass orange juice
small piece melon, diced and mixed with 2 oz
mandarins
1 cup tea or coffee, no sugar

Lunch: 2 oz shredded cabbage, 2 oz carrots, 2 oz chopped
peppers, sprinkled with lemon juice and parsley
½ avocado pear
1 cup tea or coffee, no sugar

Dinner: 1 pork or lamb chop, grilled
                   ½ jacket potato sprinkled with raw onion and carrot
                   1 fresh apple
                   1 cup lemon tea

Sunday

Breakfast: 1 cup peach juice
                   1 scrambled egg on 1 slice wholewheat toast
                   1 cup tea or coffee, no sugar
Mid-morning: 1 yogurt sprinkled with cinnamon, nutmeg or black
                   molasses
Lunch: Salad bowl of chopped lettuce, celery and water-
                   cress mixed with ½ cup cold meat or chicken
                   1 peach, sliced and mixed with 1 sliced apple
                   1 cup tea or coffee, no sugar
Dinner: ½ grilled grapefruit
                   2 slices roast lamb
                   ½ cup spinach
                   1 cup tea or coffee, no sugar

EXOTIC AQUARIAN RECIPES

Aquarius rules Russia and Sweden. Members of this sign will
particularly appreciate foods from these places so, when you have
put your diet aside, try the Russian menu below. (Hint for seducers:
this is a dish certain to liquefy that water carrier!)

Peasant Caviar
Beat half a pound of cottage cheese with 4 ounces of grated Edam
cheese, one small grated onion and half a teaspoon of paprika
pepper. Serve this with Salmon Mousse.

Salmon Mousse
7 oz tinned pink salmon
½ pint cream
packet aspic jelly (½ pint)
tabasco sauce
black pepper

Put fish, excluding back bones, in liquidiser with ½ pint aspic jelly
and turn it on for 1 minute. Pour into mould or dish. Stir in cream.
Add black pepper to taste and a dash of tabasco sauce. Cover with
foil, and put in refrigerator overnight. Serve with Peasant Caviar.

HOW DO YOU SHAPE UP AS AN AQUARIAN?

1. Do you feel dizzy after climbing a flight of stairs?
2. Are you tending to be more absentminded lately?
3. Have you suffered from a minor blood disorder in the last 6 months?
4. Do you believe that your firm and/or its boss is backward-thinking?
5. Do you take work home in the evenings?
6. Is it difficult for you to remember the last time you had an early night? (And I mean for sleeping purposes!)
7. Is it at least 6 months since you made love in the afternoon?
8. At present do you feel unable to cope with your partner's emotional needs?

More than 3 "Yes" answers probably mean you are an Aquarian on the way to overweight and health problems, and it's a good bet you are difficult—if not downright impossible—to live with right now.

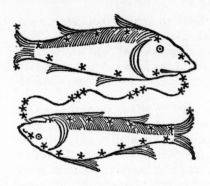

Pisces (the fish)
The sign of the poet or interpreter

February 20—March 20

The third water sign: Kind, retiring, gentle, sensitive, unlucky, often moody, indecisive
Ruler: Neptune   **Gems:** Chrysolite, moonstone
Colour: Sea green   **Metal:** Tin

GENERAL CHARACTERISTICS

Pisceans are considerate, sensitive and intuitive. They are observant in very subtle ways, and are often psychic. They have vivid imaginations and are suggestible and impressionable. In weaker types this may take the form of illusions and delusions, and in order to preserve them these subjects are inclined to indulge in drugs or alcohol; they are also likely to be dreamy and impractical, or detrimentally emotional. There is a tremendous difference between the positive and the negative Piscean, the one being able to rise to the top in every field, the other being at the very depths of degradation and despair. When Pisceans have to choose between common sense and theoretical idealism they use down-to-earth methods. They usually manage to have all the material trappings of comfort. If however there is a discrepancy between their ideals and the realities of their life then they can become restless and discontented. They are sympathetic to others, but are usually modest and unassuming and lack confidence in themselves. They have agreeable natures, are quite domesticated, and are often so pleasant they are inevitably the pet of the family. Weak types tend to be lazy and attached to the home because it is the most comfortable place to be.

Pisceans have to fight hard for stability and to resist the impulse of the moment. They are extraordinarily pliable and adaptable. They are not concerned with superficial appearance, more with the inner being. To them there is little difference between the reality and the dream. They can write and speak fluently; but there is not much worldly ambition in Neptune people. Most of them don't give a fig for rank, power or leadership, and wealth holds little attraction. Pisceans' charm of manner and good nature impress most people. Those of this sign are indifferent to insults, recriminations and others' opinions, though of course the Fish is not totally bland. This type does have a temper when finally aroused and then can be bitingly sarcastic, with a clever caustic tongue. However Pisceans normally take the line of least resistance and the cool waters of Neptune continually wash away their anger. They have great compassion and a desire to help the sick and weak, like the Virgoan, but the Piscean takes the extra step of trying to understand the hearts of the burdened and friendless, the failures and the misfits; to help is their first instinct. There are Piscean business people who are crusty and brisk, but it's only a fragile shell.

The Piscean woman tends to think that her lover, brother or father—in fact any man she knows—can lick the whole world with one hand tied behind his back. It takes a surprisingly small amount to convince her, and her touching faith is part of the reason for her popularity. A short conversation with this female and a man instantly relaxes.

Famous Pisceans: Edward Albee, Harry Belafonte, Martin Bormann, Chopin, "Buffalo Bill" Cody, Albert Einstein, Edward Kennedy, Ralph Nader, Linus Pauling, Elizabeth Taylor, George Washington.

LOVE, SEX AND THE PISCEAN

It should be remembered that the Fish is sensitive, vulnerable and can be easily hurt. This individual's shyness is due to a keen and painful consciousness of his or her own limitations. Pisceans need to know that their virtues are counted by someone they admire;

encouragement should never be withheld, for this type is a learner emotionally and requires boundless reassurance, faith and affection. The Piscean female is sentimental and when her feelings are wounded will cry buckets; she'll give her heart to her children (except the large hunk she saves for her man), and the plainer, weaker or sicklier ones will have a slight edge with her. All Pisceans are soft and tender when in love and have an unequalled capacity for dedication and self-sacrifice. They do the nice things in life quietly and with so little pretence that people all too often fail to appreciate them. They know intuitively how to please and think only of giving pleasure to their loved ones, and are often taken for granted. Piscean love is pure, charming, romantic and poetic.

The Piscean man needs a very understanding woman, for on some days she'll receive much attention, frequent phone calls, love letters; then, quite suddenly and for no apparent reason, he will withdraw into his own world, locking her out. The Piscean woman needs to find a man whose imagination is on a par with her own, someone she can spoil and fuss over. But all Pisceans must be careful in their approach to emotional relationships. They can be easily carried away and discover too late that the marvellous attributes they saw in their lover do not really exist. They find it difficult to cope with the practical aspects of a relationship, yet they make wonderful lovers and have a genuine flair for the romantic.

While all members of this sign cannot be described as masochistic, they do tend to devote themselves to their partner. For the most part to be dominated excites them and makes them fully aware of their sexuality. This is reflected in the fact that many Piscean women have fantasies about rape, being forced into prostitution or some other degradation, although of course in reality this would sicken them. Similarly, the Piscean man dreams of wifeswapping, but given the right circumstances would probably run a mile. Pisceans are highly sexed, pliable but extremely sensitive.

FASHION AND THE PISCEAN

Pisces woman is delightfully vague and dreamy and without knowing a thing about economics manages to dress as though she were turned out by Christian Dior or Balmain. Whether wearing fluffy angora mittens in winter, dainty full skirts in spring, brief bikinis in summer or warming her hands in her boyfriend's pockets in autumn—she is eternally feminine in all seasons. Everything that is pretty and delicate will appeal to her. She could be described as a charmingly overgrown Shirley Temple; men can't resist her. Pisceans have extraordinarily beautiful fine hair, and this type will tend to wear it in styles featuring waves and curls, ribbons and headbands.

But add a few years—say twenty—to our Shirley Temple, plus something like a hundred pounds and what do you have? The return of Baby Jane—hideous! So, my Piscean friends, at the risk of injuring those sensitive feelings let me tentatively suggest that once you lose that elfin figure you adjust your wardrobe. Try hard to resist those bows, frills and sweet little flowers; they'll do absolutely nothing for you, I promise you, until you melt away those pounds of fat. Pastel pinks, blues and yellows are all very well, but right now not all together, please. Dress in one colour. Choose a loose style and an outfit minus all those bits and bobs. Your famous Piscean eyes can be given that little bit extra make-up, and this together with your lovely hair should be enough to ensure you a reasonable number of compliments over the next few weeks.

PHYSICAL CHARACTERISTICS AND HEALTH

The Piscean man tends to have a slim, graceful, straight body; fine, silky hair; a pale face, with a dimple or two; light, sad eyes; possibly large ears.

The Piscean woman generally has a very feminine shape, with a heavy bust, and rather thick limbs; soft hair and skin; thick eyebrows and expressive eyes.

Pisceans' feet are often quite noticeable: either very small and dainty, including the men's; or else huge and spread out, like a tired washerwoman's. Similarly their hands will either be tiny and fragile or big-boned with the appearance of belonging behind a plough. The skin is soft, the hair is fine, often wavy and usually light. Piscean eyes are heavy-lidded and full of strange, enigmatic lights. They may be slightly protruding, they are always extremely compelling, or simply beautiful. The features are elastic and mobile, and they usually sport more dimples than wrinkles. Pisceans are tall, sometimes awkwardly built but with extraordinary grace; they positively seem to flow along instead of walking, as if swimming across the room or down the street.

These types tend to think they can live forever and act accordingly. The Fish typically doesn't take good care of himself or herself. Chances are Pisceans spend too much energy—and they don't have much to spare—helping relatives in trouble or taking on the burdens of a friend. Both emotional and financial problems can be a serious strain on Pisceans' health, which is rarely robust to begin with, so Pisceans must conserve themselves and refrain from succumbing to stimulants or sedatives, fatigue and other people's emergencies. Weak as infants, seldom sturdy as children, Pisceans tend to have a slow metabolism, which is why they often wake up sleepy-eyed and listless.

Poor eating habits can bring troubles with liver and intestinal functions and digestive disorders; colds, 'flu and pneumonia may also plague Pisceans. This sign rules the feet, and many of its subjects suffer from fallen arches. However, these individuals have a hidden resistance, and one of the challenges of Neptune is to discover this latent strength and call on it. Pisceans can literally hypnotise themselves into or out of anything they choose, be it fear of cats, spiders, heights, confined places or flying. Although this sign can be somewhat frail in health, if Pisces subjects are well balanced and their activities are wisely guided then they can enjoy excellent health.

CAUSES OF PISCEAN OBESITY AND HOW TO COPE

Pisces is another characteristically thin sign, and the exceptions to the rule can blame alcohol or liquid in general for their plumpness but rarely food. Many born under this sign develop the habit of a dozen cups of tea or coffee a day, hankering for soda pop, or a yen for something stronger. However, because of their tendency to go to extremes, they are advised to leave liquor quite alone although it brings them enticing relief. It lulls them pleasantly with a false sense of security, but it's a dangerous lullaby. Of course not every Piscean who drinks a glass of gin a week becomes an alcoholic, but the percentage is higher than it really ought to be. Most Pisceans are indecisive and secretive, not easy traits for others to live with. But nagging and bullying often result in our poetic friend becoming a secret drinker in an effort to forget his or her problems. If only Pisceans could bring themselves to discuss their worries more openly then some of the tension in their lives could be relieved and the cork put back firmly in the bottle. It's pressure Pisceans cannot stand and pressure is the first thing to drive them to keeping a secret drinks supply. Those in this individual's immediate vicinity can therefore be of great assistance: they should not impinge on the Piscean's private thoughts nor try to change this irresponsible character. It will be to no avail anyway. This type will be unimpressed by the fact that the gas bill needs paying, especially if the present mood is one of escapism. Pisceans should find an outlet for their natural creative talents; it's not being suggested that they're all inhibited or suppressed Van Goghs or Cézannes but they certainly need some way of participating in an artistic pursuit and should be encouraged in that direction.

Generally speaking Pisceans who have forsaken their typical slim silhouette are living a far too mundane life or with an incompatible partner; so some sort of new hobby could be invaluable. It's far better than turning to escapism through drink or drugs, and it doesn't harm the waistline.

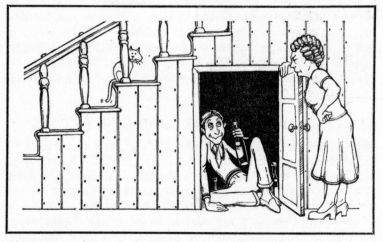

The Piscean takes to the bottle when feeling threatened

WHAT KIND OF DIET?

Most Pisceans suffer from a deficiency of iron. Plants and vegetables take in the organic iron element from the soil and carry it to the leaves where it is formed into chlorophyll, the green colouring matter of nature. It is the iron and chlorophyll, which form the haemoglobin of the red corpuscles of the blood. Without iron the function of breathing would have no physiological value and metabolism could not take place, and there would be no assimilation of nutrients from digested food. Deficiency of iron in the system can result in ailments such as low blood pressure, anaemia, inflammation, gastritis, neuritis, piles. Foods containing iron are of greater value if eaten raw, since cooking tends to destroy the iron content; if they must be heated, cook them conservatively and ensure they are not overcooked. Pisceans are lucky in having a large range of foods with this mineral to choose from to include in their diet: peas, beans, green leafy vegetables such as spinach and lettuce, dried fruits such as raisins, dates, figs and prunes, nuts, cereals, root vegetables and all fresh fruit, black molasses, liver, turnip greens, wheatgerm, kidney, beet tops, apricots, dandelions, whole-wheat bread. A conscientious Piscean will eat generously from this range, which will do much to improve that spotty skin and worn out feeling.

SPECIAL PISCEAN RECIPES

Fresh Fruit Salad
Cut some oranges in half and remove the pulp, leaving the orange peel cups intact. Shred a pineapple, cut up the pulp of the oranges and mix with some seedless raisins. Fill the orange peels cups and dress with a small amount of whipped cream.

Piscean Casserole
Take 1 or 2 carrots, $\frac{1}{2}$ a small swede or turnip, $\frac{1}{2}$ cupful soaked peas, $\frac{1}{2}$ onion, $\frac{1}{2}$ oz butter, and seasoning; prepare the vegetables and cut into small pieces. Brown the onion in a little butter then place all the ingredients in a casserole with the melted butter and $\frac{1}{2}$ cup water. Let simmer until quite tender.

Piscean Salad
Grate 1 small swede and 1 large carrot into separate heaps; arrange these on lettuce leaves and sliced celery and onion. Sprinkle with a little grated cheese and serve with mayonnaise.

Dried Fruit Salad
Chop figs, prunes, apricots and dates into small pieces and soak overnight in sufficient water to which has been added the juice of an orange or lemon. Serve fruit in the juice.

Piscean Paste
Mince $\frac{1}{2}$ cup dates, $\frac{1}{2}$ cup ground nuts, and mix well to make a paste, to which should be added a teaspoonful of finely grated lemon peel. Add a little lemon juice if desired; spread on whole-meal or rye bread.

THE SEVEN DAY PISCEAN DIET

Monday

Breakfast:	1 glass pear juice
	1 slice wholemeal or rye bread, spread with thin layer Piscean Paste
	1 cup black coffee
Lunch:	½ oz sweetcorn
	¼ head cabbage
	2 celery sticks
	1 medium onion, sliced
	½ cup diced cold lean meat
	1 yogurt with dessertspoonful brewers' yeast
	1 cup lemon tea
Dinner:	Piscean Casserole
	1 slice wholemeal bread
	dried fruit salad
	1 cup tea or coffee, no sugar

Tuesday

Breakfast:	1 glass pineapple juice
	2 apricots filled with fruit cocktail
	1 slice rye toast
	1 cup black coffee
Lunch:	Small cheese or spinach soufflé
	small jacket potato, with 2 oz grated cheese
	1 glass tomato juice
Dinner:	3 oz lean meat (approx 2 slices)
	Piscean Salad
	1 cup strawberries or loganberries
	1 cup tea or coffee, no sugar

Wednesday

Breakfast:	1 glass orange or lemon juice
	4 oz grapes chopped and mixed with whole walnuts
	1 cup black coffee
Lunch:	1 slice cheese on rye toast
	1 yogurt sprinkled with cinnamon
	1 cup lemon tea
Dinner:	1 plate lentil or pea soup
	1 small jacket potato filled with scrambled egg

1 slice wholemeal bread
fresh fruit salad
1 cup tea or coffee, no sugar

Thursday

Breakfast: 1 glass pear juice
1 cup dried fruit salad
1 slice wholemeal toast
1 cup black coffee

Lunch: Medium portion any saltwater fish
½ cup spinach
1 sliced tomato with some radishes
1 glass buttermilk

Dinner: ½ green pepper filled with 3 oz minced beef and
onion, sprinkled with grated Cheddar cheese
small green salad sprinkled with lemon juice
1 baked banana with brown sugar
1 cup lemon tea

Friday

Breakfast: 1 glass pineapple juice
½ cup stewed prunes or figs
1 slice rye toast, with ½ oz butter
1 cup black coffee

Lunch: 2 slices lean meat
½ cup cauliflower
½ cup fresh green peas or green leafy vegetable
½ cup green beans
1 apple, orange or pear
1 cup lemon tea

Dinner: Medium portion white fish sprinkled with parsley
and lemon juice
½ cup dried peas
½ cup root vegetable
1 yogurt sprinkled with raisins
1 cup black coffee

Saturday

Breakfast: 1 glass pure orange or lemon juice
small bowl cereal sprinkled with 1 oz hazelnuts
1 cup black coffee

Lunch: Medium portion liver
                   1 rasher grilled bacon
                   2 boiled potatoes
                   ½ cup green beans
                   small bowl fresh fruit salad/dried fruit salad
                   1 cup tea or coffee, no sugar
Dinner: Medium portion lean meat or fish
                   ½ cup green leafy vegetable
                   ½ cup fresh peas
                   1 yogurt sprinkled with cinnamon
                   1 cup lemon tea

Sunday

Breakfast: 1 glass pineapple or orange juice
                   2 lamb's kidneys
                   1 slice wholemeal or rye bread
                   1 cup tea or coffee, no sugar
Lunch: 2 slices roast meat
                   2 boiled potatoes, no butter
                   ½ cup turnip greens or spinach
                   1 yogurt with wheatgerm
                   1 cup lemon tea
Dinner: Medium portion liver or 2 slices lean poultry
                   Piscean Salad
                   ½ cup apricots, prunes or 2 oz dates
                   1 cup café-au-lait

EXOTIC PISCEAN RECIPE

Pisces rules Portgual, Sudan and Normandy and food from these
places will be particularly enjoyed by the Piscean. The following
dish from Normandy is therefore well worth a try after your diet.
(Hint to seducers: this dish will get the silvery fish turned on swim-
mingly!)

Sole en Matelote à la Normande (Sole stewed in cider with mussels)
1 lb fine fat sole
2 pints of mussels
1 wineglass of dry cider
1 large onion
seasoning

1 tablespoon butter
1 tablespoon parsley butter

Slice the onion finely and melt it in the butter, stewing it very gently until it is quite soft but still pale yellow. Meanwhile put the cleaned mussels in a saucepan with the cider, set them over a fast flame and extract them as soon as they open.

Put the onion mixture, well seasoned, into a long shallow fire-proof dish; on top place the sole, skinned on both sides. Through a muslin pour into it enough stock from the mussels to barely cover it. Cover the dish, and cook in a moderate oven for 15 minutes. Put the shelled mussels round the fish and the parsley butter on top of it. Return to the oven for 5 minutes, just sufficient time to allow the mussels to heat through. Serve in the same dish.

Be sure to use a porcelain or enamel-lined dish; tin or cast-iron will turn the cider black.

A small whole turbot, a sea-bream, a piece of skate, or fillets of John Dory (St Pierre) can be cooked in the same way.

HOW DO YOU SHAPE UP AS A PISCEAN?

1. Is it becoming increasingly difficult for you to make decisions?
2. Do you need a drink as soon as you arrive home from work?
3. Do you feel the need to be alone more often than usual lately?
4. Do you smoke more than 15 cigarettes a day?
5. Do you worry about fading attractions?
6. Do you feel that the romance has gone out of your life?
7. Do you often drink alone?
8. Have you recently tended to disregard your partner's feelings about making love?

More than 3 "Yes" answers to the above indicate that you are a Piscean on the way to overweight and health problems too, and what's more you are becoming a real pain in the neck!

EXERCISE AND THE BODY

Each sign rules a part of the body, that part being more vulnerable than normal for those born under the sign associated with it.
Aries rules *the head and face.*
Taurus rules *the throat, neck, ears and jaw.*
Gemini rules *the arms, hands, shoulders, lungs.*
Cancer rules *the chest and stomach.*
Leo rules *the heart, spine, back.*
Virgo rules *the abdomen and intestines.*
Libra rules *the kidneys and lower back.*
Scorpio rules *the genitals, bladder and gall bladder.*
Sagittarius rules *the hips and thighs.*
Capricorn rules *the bones, joints, knees.*
Aquarius rules *the calves, ankles, blood circulation.*
Pisces rules *the feet.*

A certain amount of regular exercise is always beneficial in combination with the correct diet, and the following exercises have been categorised according to the parts of the body they affect most. Once you have identified the areas of your figure that need toning up, work out a moderate daily routine incorporating the appropriate exercises.

Face
★ Rest elbows on table then tuck both thumbs under tip of chin-bone, first two fingers of each hand touching temples. Gently and slowly open mouth letting lower jaw "fight" hard against thumbs (you'll be able to feel the facial muscles working). Relax and repeat.
★ With elbows still on table, rest fingertips over closed eyelids, then very gently and slowly attempt to screw up eyes but let your fingers stop you. Repeated 3 times a day this will tone the eye-area muscles.
★ To help tone away over-chubby cheeks or a double chin (in private) simply say: "Oooh! Eeek!" in a tick-tock rhythm, making mouth first as round then as wide as it will go.

Chin and jaw
★ Close mouth and pull corners downwards hard. Hold for a count of 6; relax.
★ Slowly (in private!) stick tongue out to fullest extent, then bend it up as if to touch your nose so that you feel under-chin area being braced. Repeat 3 times.

Neck
★ Let neck go limp and, completely relaxed, slowly roll head full circle once in each direction.
★ Sit upright with relaxed shoulders. Keeping shoulders still, look over right shoulder, then left, switching in a tick-tock rhythm and swivelling in each direction as far as possible, 5 times. To the same rhythm, now drop head as far forward as you can, then lift and stretch it as far back as it will go, keeping shoulders down throughout.
★ Move right ear down as if trying to touch right shoulder with it, but don't let shoulder rise. Alternating with left ear to left shoulder, repeat 3 times.

Shoulders
★ Sit comfortably, back straight. Raising right shoulder try to touch right ear with it; relax. Repeat with left shoulder.
★ Pick up an object such as a book and with one hand pass it over your back to other hand. Repeat, changing hands. This will keep shoulders supple and free from stiffness which could hinder hand and arm movements.

Heart and lungs
★ Stand erect, arms at sides. Begin running on the spot, raising each foot at least 4 inches and lifting knees forward. After 50 steps, do 10 hops with both feet leaving floor together. This exercise is primarily to condition heart and lungs, but will also benefit legs.

Bustline
★ Sitting before a small suitcase or typewriter, press sides of case with hands, arms outstretched. Hold for a count of 6, then relax. Repeat.
★ Sitting or standing comfortably, bring your hands up in front of you and grab left wrist with right hand, right wrist with left. Without moving hands, push sharply (you should feel your breasts perking up), hold for a count of 6; relax.
★ Stand comfortably, arms by sides. Very slowly raise arms sideways to a point halfway between shoulders and head. Now slowly draw arms forward, consciously using pectoral muscles (situated slightly above and to one side of each breast). Stop before arms touch, and pull shoulderblades together towards your spine, thus forcing your arms apart and to the sides. Slowly lower your arms and relax muscles.

Tops of arms and bustline
★ Let your arms hang at sides then slowly bring them both up behind your back and put the palms together. Hold for a count of 5; relax, and repeat.

Upper arms
★ Stand with back to a wall, about 9 inches (23 cm) away from it Press palms flat against it. Hold for a count of 6, then relax. Repeat.

Stomach
★ Lie on your back, feet hooked under a heavy piece of furniture. Sit up slowly without using your hands. Repeat.
★ In any odd moments, whether standing or lying down, pull stomach in and up, hold for a count of 6; relax, and repeat. Will help keep muscles of stomach flat.

Waist
★ Lie down with arms at sides. Slowly bring your knees up to your chest. Slowly straighten your legs without them touching floor. Relax and repeat.
★ Stand up straight with feet slightly apart. With hands on hips twist your body, keeping hips still. Move waist from side to side.

Waistline and midriff
★ Stand with feet apart; loosely swing your body down from the waist only. Swing to the left, the right, then up to standing position again. Repeat.

Waist, midriff and hips
★ Lying on your back on the bed, draw your knees up into the air so that soles of feet are flat on bed. Without lifting feet or body, swing knees over as far as possible to the left and over as far as possible to the right. Repeat.

Hips
★ Extending arms above your head, swing head and shoulders sideways from left to right and back again, like a windscreen-wiper. This will help to loosen the hips.

Hips and bottom
★ Kneel and fold your arms in front of you. Sit on the floor, on your right side; lift yourself up and sit on the left. Repeat.
★ Stand straight and hold the back of a chair for support. Bend

your knees; hold when you are halfway down, then continue to a squatting position. Hold, then slowly stand, stopping again halfway up. Repeat.

Buttocks

★ Knock buttocks against a hard wall, up to 50 times each side every night.

★ While sitting, clench buttock muscles tightly, hold for count of 6, relax. Repeat ad lib.

Buttocks, back and thighs

★ Lie face down, arms along sides, hands under thighs, palms pressing against thighs. Raise head, shoulders and left leg as high as possible from floor, keeping leg straight. Lower to floor. Repeat, raising head, shoulders and right leg. Continue by alternating legs.

Thighs

★ Whenever climbing a flight of stairs, straighten each leg fully with each step.

★ While waiting for a kettle to boil, stand with feet about 20 inches apart, toes turned out. Keeping heels on the ground, bend knees as far as possible over toes, then snap up straight. Repeat, keeping back straight.

★ Sit on floor, holding the soles of your feet together, then rock from side to side.

★ Lie on side, legs straight, lower arm stretched over head along floor, top arm used for balance. Raise upper leg 18 to 24 inches. Lower to starting position. Repeat; roll to other side and start again.

Knees

★ When picking something up, instead of just leaning forward, keep the upper part of your body upright and flex your knees to get down.

Legs, feet and toes

★ Spend a few minutes each day walking about the house on tiptoe. This will benefit the whole of the leg.

Feet and ankles

★ Sit on floor, legs straight and about 6 inches apart, hands behind body for support, feet relaxed. Press toes away from body as far as possible. Bring toes towards body, hooking feet as much as possible; relax and repeat.

⋆ Sit on floor, legs straight and heels 14 inches apart, hands behind body for support, feet relaxed. Move feet so that toes make large circular movements. Press out and around and in and towards the body. Move toes in one direction some of the time and then reverse the direction.

⋆ Stand erect, arms at sides, feet about 12 inches apart. First raise up on to toes, then lower until feet are flat on floor. Next roll outward on sides of feet, then roll feet so that outside edge of foot is off floor. Return to starting position. Repeat.

Feet and toes
⋆ Take off your shoes and try to pick up any small object with your toes.

Whole body
⋆ Standing behind a chair, swing one leg from left to right over the chair back, then from right to left, keeping the leg straight. Repeat with the other leg.

Posture
⋆ Sit on floor, knees bent, feet on floor, hands clasped about knees, head bent forward and body relaxed. Straighten body and lift head to look directly ahead. Pull in muscles of abdomen. Relax to starting position. Repeat.

⋆ Lie on back, knees bent, feet on floor, arms slightly to side. Relax muscles of trunk. Press lower part of back to floor by tightening muscles of abdomen and back. Relax to starting position. Repeat.

⋆ Lie on back, legs straight and together, arms slightly to side. Relax muscles of trunk. Press lower part of back to floor by tightening muscles of abdomen and back. Relax to starting position. Repeat.

Good posture will help you make the most of your figure, whatever stage of your diet you have reached.

CALORIE EXPENDITURE

Sedentary activities—80-100 calories per hour:
Eating; reading; writing; listening to radio; watching television; sewing; typing; playing cards; office desk work.

Light activities—110-160 calories per hour:
Dusting; cooking; washing dishes; ironing; walking slowly; standing.

Moderate activities—170-240 calories per hour:
Making beds; mopping; gardening; light carpentry; walking moderately fast; activities with vigorous arm movements.

Vigorous activities—230-350 calories per hour:
Heavy scrubbing; handwashing large clothing; golfing; walking fast.

Strenuous activities—350 or more calories per hour:
Playing tennis; swimming; running; bicycling; dancing; ski-ing; playing football.

CALORIE TABLE

Food	Measures	Calories
Almonds	8 nuts	100
Apples, baked	1 large with 2 tablespoons sugar	200
fresh	1 medium	50
stewed	3 tablespoons	120
Apple sauce, sweetened	½ cup	100
Apricots, canned in syrup	3 halves with 2 tablespoons juice	110
dried, raw	6 halves	160
fresh	3 medium	30
Asparagus	5 medium stalks	15
Avocado pear	½ medium (about 4 inches long)	110
Bacon, back, fried	3 medium rashers	330
gammon, fried	1 thick rasher	380
streaky, fried	3 rashers	300
Bacon fat	1 tablespoon	100
Beans, broad, boiled	½ cup	100
butter, boiled	½ cup	130
canned with pork	½ cup	160
dried	½ cup cooked	130
lima	½ cup	100
Beef, corned	1 slice about 1 inch thick	100
dried	2 thin slices	50
hamburger steak	1 patty (4 to 5 per pound)	150
round, lean	1 medium slice (2 ounces)	100
sirloin, roast	1 medium slice (3 ounces)	150
steak, grilled	1 medium	320
tongue	2 slices	50
Beetroot	2 beets (2 inches in diameter)	50
Biscuits, baking powder	2 small	100
cream crackers	2 biscuits	70
digestive	2 biscuits	130
rusks	2 medium	100
sweet	2 medium	130
water	2 biscuits	100
Blackberries, fresh	1 cup	100
Blueberries, fresh	1 cup	90
Bread, rye	1 medium slice (¼ inch thick)	75
white	1 medium slice	75
white	1 thin slice	55
wholewheat	1 medium slice	75
Broccoli	4 medium stalks	20
Brussels sprouts, boiled	6 small sprouts	50
Butter	2 small pats (1 tablespoonful)	100
Cabbage, boiled	1 cup	50
Cake, angel	1 medium slice	160
chocolate or vanilla sponge	1 medium slice (not iced)	180
cup cake with icing	1 medium	250

Food	Measures	Calories
fruit cake (Dundee type)	1 slice	300
Cantaloupe melon	½ medium	50
Carrots	3 medium	25
Cashewnuts	4 nuts	100
Cauliflower, boiled	½ small head	25
Caviar	½ tablespoonful	30
Celery	3 stalks	15
Cheese, Camembert	1 medium piece (1 ounce)	90
Cheddar	1 medium piece	120
cottage	5 tablespoons	100
cream	½ tablespoon	90
Edam	1 medium piece	90
Gorgonzola	1 medium piece	115
Parmesan, grated	1 tablespoon	100
Stilton	1 medium piece	140
Cherries, canned	3 tablespoons	125
fresh, sweet	15 large	75
Chestnuts	4 shelled	30
Chicken, boiled	½ medium broiler	250
roast	1 medium slice	100
Chocolate, fudge	1 piece (1 inch square)	120
mints	1 mint (1½ inch diameter)	100
milk	1 small bar	250
plain	1 small bar	240
unsweetened	1 square	100
Clams	6 rounds	100
Cocoa, unsweetened	1 cup made with ½ milk	150
Coconut, desiccated	2 tablespoons	100
Cod liver oil	1 tablespoon	100
Cod steak	1 medium	150
Coffee	1 cup (1 tablespoon milk, no sugar)	30
Cola-type soft drinks	1 glass (6 ounce bottle)	75
Cooking fats, vegetable	1 tablespoon	100
Corn, canned	½ cup	100
Cornflakes	1 cup	80
Cornmeal	1 tablespoon uncooked	35
Cornstarch pudding	½ cup	200
Crab meat	2 tablespoons	100
Cream, light (single)	1 tablespoon	40
heavy (double)	1 tablespoon	80
whipped	3 tablespoons	100
Cucumber	½ medium	10
Currants, black or red, stewed	3 tablespoons	80
dried	1 tablespoon	70
Custard, boiled or baked	½ cup	130
Damsons, stewed	3 tablespoons	120
Dates	4	100
Duck, roast	1 medium thick slice	200
Egg, boiled or raw	1 medium	75
fried	1 egg	140

Food	*Measures*	*Calories*
omelette or soufflé	2 eggs	200
poached	1 egg	75
scrambled	1 tablespoon	200
Endive, raw	medium serving	10
Figs, dried	3 small	100
green	2 medium	50
Flour, white or wholegrain	1 tablespoon unsifted	50
Frankfurter	1 sausage	100
Fruit salad, canned or stewed	3 tablespoons	70
Fruit squashes or cordials	1 glass diluted	50
Gelatin, fruit flavoured	3 ounces unprepared	330
ready to serve	½ cup	85
Ginger ale	1 cup	85
Gingerbread	2 inch square	270
Goose, roast	1 medium serving	220
Gooseberries, stewed	3 tablespoons	80
Grapefruit, fresh	½ medium	20
canned	3 tablespoons	60
Grapefruit juice, unsweetened	1 cup	100
Grape juice	½ cup	80
Grape nuts	¼ cup	100
Grapes, black	12 grapes	30
white	12 grapes	35
Greengages, stewed or canned	3 tablespoons	120
Haddock, smoked, steamed	1 medium fillet	110
Halibut, steamed	1 medium piece	150
Ham, lean, boiled	3 thin slices (2 ounces)	250
Herring, fried	1 medium fish	300
Honey	1 tablespoon	120
Ice cream	½ cup	200
Ice-cream soda	fountain size	325
Jellies and jams	1 rounded tablespoon	100
Kale	½ cup	50
Kidney, lamb, fried	3 medium	200
Kipper, grilled	pair of medium	200
Lamb, chop, grilled	1 medium	250
roast	1 medium slice	100
Lard	1 tablespoon	100
Lemon, fresh	1 medium	8
Lemon juice	1 tablespoon	5
Lentils, boiled	2 tablespoons	100
Lettuce	2 large leaves	5
Lime juice cordial	1 glass diluted	40
Liver	1 medium slice	100
Liverwurst	1 slice (½ inch thick)	100
Lobster meat	1 cup	150

Food	Measures	Calories
Macaroni	¾ cup cooked	130
Mackerel, fried	1 medium	200
Mandarins, canned	3 tablespoons	150
Maple syrup	1 tablespoon	70
Margarine	1 tablespoon	100
Marshmallow	1 small	20
Mayonnaise, home made	1 tablespoon	80
Melon	1 medium slice	30
Milk, fresh, whole	1 cup	170
buttermilk	1 cup	85
condensed, sweetened	1½ tablespoons	100
skimmed, dried	2½ tablespoons	100
skimmed, fresh	1 cup	85
Mincemeat	1 tablespoon	70
Mineral waters	1 glass	90
Mints, cream	½ inch cube	5
Muffins, bran	1 medium	90
1-egg	1 medium	130
Mushrooms	10 large	10
fried	medium helping (2 ounces)	125
Mussels	15	60
Nectarines	1 medium	40
Noodles	¾ cup cooked	130
Oatmeal	¾ cup cooked	130
Oil (corn, cottonseed, olive, groundnut)	1 tablespoon	100
Okra	10-15 pods	50
Olives	6 medium	40
Onions	4 medium	100
fried	medium portion (1½ ounces)	150
Orange, fresh	1 medium	50
juice	1 cup	120
Oysters	6	40
Parsnips	3 tablespoons	50
Peaches, canned in syrup	2 halves with 3 tablespoons juice	150
dried	4 halves	100
fresh	1 medium	50
Peanuts	10 nuts	100
Peanut butter	1 tablespoon	150
Pears, canned in syrup	3 halves with 3 tablespoons juice	150
fresh	1 medium	50
Peas, canned	½ cup	65
fresh, boiled	¾ cup	100
Pecans	6 nuts	100
Pepper, green	1 medium	20
Pickles, cucumber, sour, dill	10 medium slices	10
sweet	1 small	10
Pies, apple	3 inch sector (from 9 inch pie)	200
lemon meringue	3 inch sector	300

Food	*Measures*	*Calories*
mincemeat	3 inch sector	300
pumpkin	3 inch sector	250
Pilchards, canned	2 large	200
Pineapple, canned, unsweetened	1 ½-inch slice with 1 tablespoon juice	50
fresh	1 slice (¾ inch thick)	50
juice, unsweetened	1 cup	130
Plaice, fried	1 medium	200
steamed	1 medium	100
Plums, canned	2 medium with 1 tablespoon juice	100
fresh	2 medium	50
Popcorn	1½ cups popped	100
Pork chop, lean, grilled	1 medium	250
Potato, baked (including skin)	1 medium	80
boiled	2 small or 1 medium	100
chips, fried	10 large	300
mashed	½ cup	100
roast	2 small	140
sweet	½ medium	100
Potato salad with mayonnaise	½ cup	200
Prawns	12, shelled	80
Prune juice	½ cup	100
Prunes, dried	4 medium	100
stewed	2 tablespoons	120
Pumpkin	medium portion	40
Radishes	5	10
Raisins, dried	¼ cup	90
Raspberries, fresh	1 cup	90
stewed, canned	3 tablespoons	150
Rhubarb, stewed and sweetened	½ cup	100
Rice, boiled	¾ cup	130
Salad dressing, boiled	1 tablespoon	25
French	1 tablespoon	90
mayonnaise	1 tablespoon	100
Salmon, canned	½ cup	110
fresh, steamed	1 medium steak	180
Sardines, drained	5 small fish	170
Sauces, bread	1 tablespoon	25
cheese	1 tablespoon	50
tartare	1 tablespoon	80
tomato	1 tablespoon	20
Sausage, pork, fried	2 large	280
rolls	1 large	250
Shrimps	24 medium	100
Sole, fried	1 medium	320
steamed	1 medium	90
Spaghetti	¾ cup cooked	130
Spinach	½ cup cooked	20
Strawberries, fresh	6 large	30
Sugar, all kinds	1 tablespoon	110
Sultanas, dried	1 tablespoon	70

Food	Measures	Calories
Sweetbreads	1 pair medium	240
Syrup, golden	1 tablespoon	100
Tangerines	1 medium	30
Tapioca, uncooked	1 tablespoon	50
Tea	1 cup (1 tablespoon milk, no sugar)	20
Tomato juice, unsweetened	1 cup	60
Tomatoes, canned	½ cup	25
fresh	1 medium	10
fried	medium portion (4 ounces)	80
Trout, steamed	1 medium	150
Tuna fish, canned	¼ cup, drained	100
Turkey, lean, roast	2 thin slices (3 ounces)	100
Turnip	1 medium	25
Veal, roast	1 medium slice (2 ounces)	130
Veal cutlet, fried	1 medium	190
Walnuts	8	100
Watercress	½ bunch	5
Watermelon	1 large slice	90
Wheatflakes	¾ cup	100
Wheatgerm	1 tablespoon	25
Wheat, shredded	1 biscuit	100
Whelks	10 medium	80
Whitebait, fried	3 heaped tablespoons	300
Whiting, fried	1 medium fillet (5 ounces)	250
steamed	1 medium fillet	100
Winkles	12	30
Yeast, brewers', dried	1 ounce	100
fresh	1 ounce	25
extract	1 ounce	40
Yogurt, natural	½ cup	150

Alcoholic beverages	Measures	Calories
Cider, dry	1 cup (½ pint)	100
sweet	½ pint	120
vintage	½ pint	180
Beer	½ pint	80-120
Brandy	1½ ounces	150
Gin	1½ ounces	150
Rum	1½ ounces	150
Whisky	1½ ounces	150
Wines, champagne	1 glass	120
port	1 small wineglass (3 ounces)	130
sherry	1 sherry glass (about 2 ounces)	75
table, red or white	1 glass (4 ounces)	90-100

Measures
1 cup = 8 ounces
3 teaspoons = 1 tablespoon
4 tablespoons = ¼ cup